Praise for *The Single-Session practice* by Windy Dryden

An enormously helpful book.
and warmth about the prac

CW01431795

Clients can make dramatic improvements right from the start of therapy, and this is capitalised on in the single session counselling approach: harnessing client's strengths and resources to facilitate change. While the book may be particularly suited to counsellors, psychotherapists, and coaches – both qualified and in training – who favour structured and goal-oriented ways of working, it is profoundly client-centred in its ethos. The book is eminently engaging and easy to follow, taking the reader from the underlying rationale for the approach to core principles of practice and concrete examples of work. Highly recommended.
Mick Cooper, Professor of Counselling Psychology, University of Roehampton

Windy Dryden has done it again. Succinctly and clearly written, as you might expect, his book makes a formidable contribution in laying out theoretical, philosophical and ethical parameters for single-session counselling. For some clients, at the right time, single-session work is exactly what is needed. This is a timely and perfectly-pitched roadmap for setting out on that journey.
Dr Andrew Reeves, Associate Professor in the Counselling Professions and Mental Health, University of Chester

A great book that packs a lot into its 170-odd pages. This is an essential guide for anyone thinking of using SSC, whether therapist or service manager – it's all here, from what SSC is, when to use it and who to use it with to answering common objections and summarising its research base. In 20 years' time we will be wondering why it took so long for services to embrace this approach. The case studies, session transcripts and answers to the practical challenges of delivering SSC reveal Professor Dryden's massive experience as practitioner, not simply an academic. If you see yourself as client-focused in your work, you need to read this. Prepare to be challenged.
Paul Grantham, consultant clinical psychologist and Professor of Clinical Psychology, PSMedUniv

Windy Dryden is Emeritus Professor of Psychotherapeutic Studies at Goldsmith's, University of London, and a Fellow of the British Psychological Society. He has authored or edited more than 230 books. His current interests are in single-session and very brief interventions in therapy and coaching. He has run training courses in single-session counselling in the UK and abroad and has contributed to its provision in university and college counselling throughout the UK.

The Single-Session Counselling Primer

Principles and Practice

Windy Dryden

PCCS
BOOKS

First published 2020

PCCS Books Ltd
Wyastone Business Park
Wyastone Leys
Monmouth
NP25 3SR
UK

Tel +44 (0)1600 891509
contact@pccs-books.co.uk
www.pccs-books.co.uk

The Single-Session Counselling Primer: principles and practice

British Library Cataloguing in Publication Data.
A catalogue record for this book is available from the British Library

ISBN 978 1 910919 56 9

Cover design by Jason Anscomb
Printed in the UK by TJ International, Padstow

Contents

Acknowledgments

To Moshe Talmon, whose vision and courage provided the catalyst for recent developments in single-session therapy.

To Michael Hoyt and Jeff Young, for their creativity and inspirational writings on single-session therapy.

To Arnie Slive and Monte Bobele, for their groundbreaking work in walk-in counselling.

To Nicola Hurton, for her invaluable help with Chapter 16.

And fnally, to Relationships Australia Victoria, from whose website and publicity materials I have drawn in Chapter 9.

Introduction

As with other developments in counselling, single-session counselling (SSC)[1] can be traced back to Sigmund Freud. Better known for longer-term therapy, Freud was consulted by Aurelia Öhm-Kronich ('Katharina') in 1893 (Freud & Breuer, 1895) and by the famous composer Gustav Mahler in 1910 (Kuehn, 1965), while he was on holiday. Both wanted immediate help for their problems and, probably because he was on holiday, Freud offered each a one-shot consultation. According to the published reports, both deemed the session useful.

A later development focused on public demonstrations of what was, effectively, SSC. In the 1920s, Alfred Adler, who split from Freud to develop what eventually became known as Adlerian therapy, did demonstrations of SSC with children and their parents, separately and together, in his newly formed child guidance clinics. These sessions were conducted in front of a mixed professional and lay audience. Albert Ellis, founder of rational emotive behaviour therapy (REBT), was influenced by Adler, and from 1965 to 2005 did SSC with volunteer members of a largely lay audience at the institute that bore his name. These

1. In this book, I use the term 'single-session counselling' (SSC), as opposed to 'single-session therapy' (SST), 'single-session work' (SSW) and 'single-session consultations', which are synonymous terms that can also be found in the literature.

sessions were deemed helpful to the volunteers themselves and to the watching audience (Ellis & Joffe, 2002). I have continued this tradition by doing live demonstrations of the way I practise SSC in meet-up groups.[2]

Other notable developments in the history of SSC include Milton Erickson's work, much of which lasted for a single session (O'Hanlon & Hexum, 1990). Everett Shostrum's famous *Three Approaches to Psychotherapy, I, II and II* videos (Daniels, 2012) can also be seen as examples of SSC. These are the so-called Gloria films, released in 1965, where 'Gloria' was interviewed by Carl Rogers (see Burry, 2008), Fritz Perls and Albert Ellis.

However, the growing interest in SSC can perhaps be traced to the publication of *Single-Session Therapy: maximising the effect of the first (and often only) therapeutic encounter*, by Moshe Talmon (1990). Talmon, with Michael Hoyt and Robert Rosenbaum, did pioneering work on SSC in the 1980s at the public Kaiser Permanente clinic in Northern California, USA.

Hoyt and Talmon (2014) edited the proceedings of the first international symposium on SSC, held in Melbourne, Australia in 2012, entitled *Capturing the Moment: single-session therapy and walk-in services*. They were also part of the team that edited the proceedings of the second international symposium,[3] held in Banff, Canada in 2015, titled *Single-Session Therapy by Walk-In or Appointment: administrative, clinical and supervisory aspects of one-at-a-time services* (Hoyt et al, 2018).

Two of the other editors of the proceedings of the second international symposium, Arnold Slive and Monte Bobele, are pioneers in the field of walk-in therapy services (a specific form of SSC) and published their groundbreaking work in *When One Hour is All You Have: effective therapy for walk-in clients* (Slive & Bobele, 2011).

---

2. Meet-up groups are online groups that host in-person events for people with shared interests. The UKCBT group hosts my demonstrations (Dryden, 2018). This is a group for people interested in cognitive behaviour therapy and coaching, and rational emotive behaviour therapy and coaching.

3. The third international symposium was held in 2019, again in Melbourne, Australia.

This book is intended as an introduction to SSC and draws on my experience of running workshops and giving presentations on SSC, and my own practice of SSC (Dryden, 2017, 2018, 2019). It covers the ideas that underpin SSC, its practice, its dissemination and its research status. It also addresses the ambivalence felt by many counsellors towards SSC. On the one hand, they are excited by the prospect of helping clients at the point of need; on the other, they are fearful that they may be short-changing or even harming clients as a result. I hope, by the end of the book, these fears will have been allayed and the excitement will have been converted into action.

Several important points are repeated in different chapters. This is deliberate and for clarity, because they are relevant to the theme of that particular chapter. I hope readers will bear with the repetition.

Windy Dryden
London and Eastbourne, 2020

References

Burry P (2008). *Living with the 'Gloria Films': a daughter's memory.* Ross-on-Wye: PCCS Books.

Daniels D (2012). *Gloria Decoded: an application of Robert Lang's communicative approach to psychotherapy.* DPsych thesis. London: Middlesex University. http://eprints.mdx.ac.uk/9787/ (accessed 18 May 2020).

Dryden W (2019). *REBT in India: very brief therapy for problems of daily living.* Abingdon: Routledge.

Dryden W (2018). *Very Brief Therapeutic Conversations.* Abingdon: Routledge.

Dryden W (2017). *Single-Session Integrated CBT (SSI-CBT): distinctive features.* Abingdon: Routledge.

Ellis A, Joffe D (2002). A study of volunteer clients who experienced live sessions of rational emotive behavior therapy in front of a public audience. *Journal of Rational-Emotive & Cognitive-Behavior Therapy 20*: 151–158.

Freud S, Breuer J (1895). *Studien Über Hysterie.* Leipzig/Vienna: Deuticke.

Hoyt MF, Bobele M, Slive A, Young J, Talmon M (eds) (2018). *Single-Session Therapy by Walk-In or Appointment: administrative, clinical, and supervisory aspects of one-at-a-time services.* New York, NY: Routledge.

Hoyt MF, Talmon MF (eds) (2014). *Capturing the Moment: single session therapy and walk-in services.* Bethel, CT: Crown House Publishing.

Kuehn JL (1965). Encounter at Leyden: Gustav Mahler consults Sigmund Freud. *Psychoanalytic Review 52*: 345–364.

O'Hanlon WH, Hexum AL (1990). *An Uncommon Casebook: the complete clinical work of Milton H. Erickson MD.* New York, NY: WW Norton & Co.

Slive A, Bobele M (eds) (2011). *When One Hour is All You Have: effective therapy for walk-in clients.* Phoenix, AZ: Zeig, Tucker & Theisen.

Talmon M (1990). *Single-Session Therapy: maximising the effect of the first (and often only) therapeutic encounter.* San Francisco, CA: Jossey Bass.

Chapter 1
What is single-session counselling?

Overview

In this opening chapter, I will consider the question, what is single-session counselling (SSC)? Briefly, obviously, it is one single session of counselling – and that is it. But I call this the Ronseal definition of SSC.[1] The situation is a little more complicated than this, as I will explain presently. So, in this chapter, I will consider:

- how many sessions SSC might comprise
- how SSC is defined – an approach to counselling, a mindset or a mode of service delivery?

How many sessions?

There is a difference of opinion in the SSC community between what I refer to as the 'purists' and the 'pragmatists'. The purists hold that SSC is one session, and that is that – no preparation

---

1. In the mid-1990s, Ronseal, a UK company selling wood-staining products, ran an advertising campaign with the slogan, 'Ronseal – does exactly what it says on the tin'. This has entered everyday language and is now commonly used to describe something obvious. The Ronseal definition of SSC is thus: 'Single-session counselling is counselling that lasts for one session and one session only.' It therefore does not include a pre-session contact or a follow-up session.

contact, no follow-up. The pragmatists, who are in the majority, hold that both counsellor and client will purposefully try to do the necessary work in the contracted session, but further help may be offered if needed.

There are times when counselling does last for a single session. These include:

- when the client decides not to return, even though the counsellor and client have contracted for more than one session. This is known as 'SSC by default'

- when the counsellor and client have agreed in advance that the client will only have one session. This is known as 'SSC by design'. There may be several reasons for this. For example, for practical reasons, the client may only be able to attend one session, or the counsellor is only offering a single session of counselling, and the client agrees to this

- when a counsellor is demonstrating their approach to counselling at a workshop or training event and asks for a volunteer from the audience to help them. Before they begin, they stress that they will not be able to see the person again after the session, and the person knows that this is the case before they volunteer.

SSC by walk-in

SSC can occur by appointment or by walk-in. A person, couple or family[2] who walk into a service run on SSC lines will receive counselling from the outset. This contrasts with non-SSC walk-in services, where the person or family will be helped to find the best therapy pathway for their problems but no counselling is offered. When a person comes to a walk-in SSC service, they usually only attend for a single session of counselling, although there is generally nothing to stop them from walking in again at a later date for another session.

---

2. While SSC can be practised with individuals, couples, families and even groups, the focus of this book will be on SSC with individuals since a) this is my area of expertise and b) most readers are likely to be working primarily with individuals.

When SSC continues for more than one session

Moshe Talmon's seminal description (1990) of his approach to SSC includes several points of contact. The first is when the person contacts the counsellor to make an appointment for SSC. The second is when the counsellor seeks information from the person (by questionnaire or by telephone) to help the client (and the counsellor) get the most out of the face-to-face session, which is the next and primary point of contact. The final point of contact occurs later and is intended as a follow-up. Although the face-to-face session is designed to be the basis of the therapeutic work, the person sometimes gets what they are looking for from the pre-session contact (Dryden, 2017).

Talmon (1990) argued that his multi-point of contact approach was still SSC, as long as a) only the main session was face-to-face and b) no other face-to-face contact occurred within a year. However, Hoyt and colleagues (2018) subsequently described this definition as arbitrary and stated that it was used to define SSC in research studies.

One session with the possibility of more

So, there is some confusion about the nature of SSC. The current view (eg. Hoyt et al, 2018) is that SSC is a purposeful endeavour where the counsellor and client meet with the intention that one session may be sufficient, but with the understanding that more sessions may be available. This allows counsellor and client to harness the power of 'now', secure in the knowledge that more help is available later on.

One-at-a-time counselling

Michael Hoyt (2011) coined the term 'one-at-a-time counselling' (OAATC). He used it to describe counselling that takes place one session at a time. The client is encouraged to reflect on what they have learned from the session, digest this learning, act on it and let time pass before deciding whether or not to seek another session (Dryden, 2019). Counselling proceeds in this way, one session at a time, until the client has achieved what they want from the process.

With OAATC, blocks of sessions are not offered to clients as a matter of course. This means waiting times for therapy are reduced as, generally speaking, when clients are offered blocks of counselling, it creates a waiting list. Since waiting lists are becoming an increasing problem for counselling agencies, particularly those in colleges and universities, OAATC may be seen as an attractive option for those wishing to reduce waiting times and offer counselling at the point of client need, rather than at the point of service availability. (I will discuss this further in Chapter 8.)

It is important to stress that OAATC does not mean that an agency does not offer blocks of sessions or ongoing counselling. It simply means that this is not offered to all clients as a matter of course. A block of counselling or ongoing counselling may still be offered to a small number of clients if they meet specific criteria for more sessions.

Approach, mindset or mode of service delivery?

Some people refer to SSC as an 'approach' to counselling, or even as a technique. In my view, nothing can be further from the truth. In my view, SSC is not an approach to counselling. Rather, it is a mindset and a way of delivering services.

SSC is a mindset

Counselling comprises a number of traditions within which there are several different approaches. For example, I edit a series of books entitled *Cognitive Behaviour Therapy: distinctive features*. Each volume in the series deals with the distinctive features of a specific approach within the overall tradition of CBT. SSC can be practised by counsellors using any of the different approaches within the various counselling traditions. Thus, it is not an approach to counselling, and it is certainly not a technique. It is much broader than that.

Rather, SSC is *both* a mindset held by SSC practitioners *and* a way of delivering counselling services. Importantly, it is also a mindset held by the client.

The counsellor's mindset

Jeff Young (2018) has outlined several features of the counsellor's SSC mindset, which I present here. Counsellors are advised to take note of and act on the following:

1. Approach the first session as if it could be the last, irrespective of diagnosis, complexity or severity.

It makes sense for the counsellor to think that the first session with a client may be their last as there is no way that the counsellor knows for sure that the client will return for another one. From this perspective, all the client and the counsellor have is 'now'. This is the case, no matter what the problems are that the client brings. Indeed, there is some evidence that clients with complex issues benefit more from a single session of counselling provided at the point of need through a walk-in service than from help provided at the point of availability (Riemer et al, 2018).

2. Explore what each client wants to walk away with at the end of the session.

Setting a meaningful goal with the client is a central part of the SSC process. What distinguishes SSC from other modes of counselling delivery is that, in SSC, the client is asked what they want to achieve from the *session,* rather than the usual question of what they want from a *course* of counselling.

3. Negotiate and prioritise with the client what to focus on.

SSC is mainly led by the client, but there are times when the client may want to focus on something that is outside their control. Thus, it is important that the counsellor negotiates the focus of the session with the client and, if the client has more than one concern, that the two agree on the client's priority.

4. Check in at various points throughout the session to ensure the work is on track.

It is easy for both counsellor and client to move away from the agreed focus. The counsellor needs to keep this tendency in mind and take on the responsibility to return them both to that focus.

5. Identify and use the client's strengths and environmental resources.

Very little of lasting use can be achieved from the session unless the counsellor helps the client to identify and apply their own internal strengths and the resources around them as they address the agreed issue. Thus, the counsellor in SSC comes to the session actively looking for opportunities to help the client make use of internal and external strengths and resources.

6. Negotiate a 'solution' with the client.

It is important in SSC that the client takes away something meaningful from the session that they can implement to help them address their presenting issue. In this book, I will refer to this 'something meaningful' as a 'solution'. This is the bridge between the client's problem and their goal, as shown in Figure 1.1. The counsellor may discuss several possible solutions with

Figure 1.1: The 'solution' is the bridge between the problem and the goal

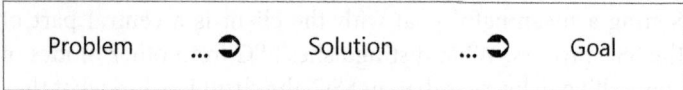

Problem	... ➲	Solution	... ➲	Goal

the client and help them select one that they (the client) thinks will work best for them and that they will be able to incorporate into their life. The counsellor will also help the client rehearse the solution in the session, if possible, so they have some experience of carrying out the solution and fine-tuning it, if necessary.

7. Help the client to develop a plan to implement the solution.

Whether or not the session will be productive for the client will depend at this point on the extent to which they implement the solution. There are two things the counsellor can do to help the client in this regard. First, the counsellor can encourage the client to develop a plan to implement the solution later, having identified and rehearsed it in the session. Second, the counsellor can help the client identify and address possible roadblocks to implementing their plan.

8. Effect closure and clarify next steps.
The counsellor in SSC keeps in mind the importance of bringing the session to a suitable conclusion, tying up any loose ends and clarifying future possibilities for the client to have more help if this is, indeed, possible. The counsellor strives to help the client leave the session with a sense of hope that they can implement the agreed solution and thereby achieve their goal, and (where this is the case) the security of knowing that more help is available and what they can do if it is not.

The client's mindset

There has been much discussion in the SSC literature about what constitutes the counsellor's mindset in SSC, but there has been little written on the mindset of the client. The power of SSC derives from the work that counsellor and client do together, and no matter how skilful the counsellor is in SSC, unless the client holds several ideas in mind that they then act on, then they will derive little lasting benefit from it. In my view, the following ideas comprise the client's optimal mindset in SSC.

1. Be ready to take care of business now.
SSC is primarily about capitalising on the moment – the time when the counsellor knows for sure that the client is 'in the room' with them and so help can be provided. If the client shares the counsellor's desire to take care of business, this is a good sign that the client will benefit from the single session.

2. Recognise that it is possible to get something meaningful from a single session of counselling, but also be realistic about what can be achieved.
The best mindset for the client in relation to SSC is a combination of *optimism* that they can derive something relevant from the process and *realism* that the change they derive will be within realistic bounds.

3. Be willing to focus on a selected problem directly.
If the client seeks counselling help and they only have one problem, then they will just focus on this one problem. However,

if they have more than one problem, they need to be able to identify, focus on and work with the problem that they want to tackle first.

4. Be prepared to take responsibility for the selected problem and to work with the counsellor to address it.

If the client takes responsibility for their target problem, then they will be able to work with the counsellor to understand it and work towards change. If they do not assume this responsibility, it is not clear what they can change.

5. See the difference between what they can and cannot control and focus on the former.

Similarly, if the client focuses on what they can change, then they will derive far more benefit from the process than if they focus more on what is outside their control. The counsellor should, if necessary, help them to make this important distinction.

6. Be willing to focus on available solutions, select the most viable and rehearse it in the session.

SSC tends to be solution-focused, and thus it is vital for the client to share this focus, be open to a variety of possible solutions, select one that seems the best on offer and be prepared to rehearse it in the session, if this is feasible.

7. Be prepared to work with the counsellor to develop a plan to implement the chosen solution.

While there is much that can be done in a single session of counselling, it is important for the client to acknowledge that the learning they derive from the session needs to be applied in their life. To aid this process, it is useful for the client to be minded to develop a plan to implement the solution that they and their counsellor have selected together.

8. Appreciate that they have strengths that they can use in the session.

When a client comes to SSC willing to identify and use their strengths to get what they want from the process, this helps them to achieve their goals.

9. Appreciate that the environment has helpful resources that they can draw on in the future.

As with internal strengths, when the client comes to SSC minded to draw on helpful resources in their environment, they will get more from the process than if they rule this out.

SSC is a way of delivering counselling services

As well as a mindset, SSC is a way of delivering services. As previously stated, it is best offered at the point of need, rather than at the point of availability. It may be accessed by appointment or by walk-in. In the latter scenario, the client is the sole arbiter of whether or not they seek help and when they seek it. SSC may be the sole service that an agency offers, but it is more common for it to sit alongside other services also offered by the agency.

Given that most clients who seek counselling from publicly funded and charitable organisations have just one session (Talmon, 1990; Hoyt & Talmon, 2014), some agencies deliberately structure their services accordingly. They make SSC the gateway service; anybody who seeks help from the agency is offered a single session, with more help available if needed. In such agencies, more than half of clients seen are satisfied with the single session at that point in their lives and given their current circumstances. The remainder are offered another appointment, ongoing counselling or a referral to one of the agencies' specialised services or those offered elsewhere (Young, 2018).

Other agencies choose not to make SSC a gateway service and prefer to offer clients the choice of whether or not to access SSC. Whichever approach is taken, SSC needs to be integrated into an agency and given sufficient resources and assistance to flourish.

Having discussed the nature of SSC, in the next chapter I will discuss why it might be used.

References

Dryden W (2019). *Single-Session 'One-At-A-Time' (OAAT) Therapy: a rational emotive behaviour therapy approach*. Abingdon: Routledge.

Dryden W (2017). *Single-Session Integrated CBT (SSI-CBT): distinctive features*. Abingdon: Routledge.

Hoyt MF (2011). Foreword. In: Slive A, Bobele M (eds). *When One Hour is All You Have: effective therapy for walk-in clients*. Phoenix, AZ: Zeig, Tucker & Theisen (ppxix-xxv).

Hoyt MF, Bobele M, Slive A, Young J, Talmon M (eds) (2018). *Single-Session Therapy by Walk-In or Appointment: administrative, clinical, and supervisory aspects of one-at-a-time services*. New York, NY: Routledge.

Hoyt MF, Talmon MF (2014). What the literature says: an annotated bibliography. In: Hoyt MF, Talmon M (eds). *Capturing the Moment: single session therapy and walk-in services*. Bethel, CT: Crown House Publishing (pp487–516).

Riemer M, Stalker CA, Dittmer L, Cait C-A, Horton S, Kermani N, Booton J (2018). The walk-in counselling model of service delivery: who benefits most? *Canadian Journal of Community Mental Health 37*: 29–47.

Talmon M (1990). *Single Session Therapy: maximising the effect of the first (and often only) therapeutic encounter*. San Francisco, CA: Jossey-Bass.

Young J (2018). SST: the misunderstood gift that keeps on giving. In: Hoyt MF, Bobele M, Slive A, Young J, Talmon M (eds) (2018). *Single-Session Therapy by Walk-In or Appointment: administrative, clinical, and supervisory aspects of one-at-a-time services*. New York, NY: Routledge (pp40–58).

Chapter 2
Why offer single-session counselling?

Overview

In this chapter, I will explain three reasons to offer SSC to clients:

- the most common number of sessions a client has is one
- people are often satisfied with a single session
- counsellors are not good at predicting how long clients will stay in counselling.

Introduction

Counsellors are trained to offer people in distress as much help as they need. In an ideal world, people in distress would get exactly that. This may be the case in the private sector, where people pay for counselling[1] out of their own pocket, but it is certainly no longer the case in the public and non-profit sectors, where the demand for counselling far outstrips the supply of counsellors employed to provide it. This is also often the case in the third sector where counsellors offer their time voluntarily.

---

1. I am using the term 'counselling' here as a generic way of referring to what are known as the 'talking therapies'.

In Britain at this time, we are seeing a new wave of understanding shown to people experiencing issues where their mental wellbeing has been compromised. We have mental health awareness days, with celebrities and members of the Royal Family coming forward to say that they have experienced psychological difficulties, challenging the shame so often attached to this. We are encouraged to come forward to seek help for our problematic responses to life's adversities, and this, from one perspective, is a wholly good thing. On the other hand, it is not a good thing if, having been encouraged to seek help, the help is not readily available to us and, in some cases, we have to wait so long that it might as well not be available at all.

The three rationales for SSC

Although, as mentioned above, counsellors are trained to help people for as long as they need such help, it depends on who is making that judgement call. For example, research tells us that therapists tend to think that clients need more psychological help than clients do themselves (eg. Maluccio, 1979). This leads us to the first rationale for SSC being offered to clients.

Internationally, the modal[2] number of sessions clients have is one

At my training workshops and presentations on SSC, I ask people to guess the modal number of counselling sessions that clients have worldwide. I make it clear that I am talking about counselling provided in the public and non-profit sectors, not in the private sector, as we don't have these data. People who do not already know the answer to this question are amazed to learn that it is one, followed by two, followed by three and so on. For example, Brown and Jones (2005) looked at a sample of 9,608 adults covered by PacifiCare Behavioral Health, a managed behavioural health care organisation in the US. They found that, among those who had therapy between 1 January 1999 and 1 September 2003, the modal number of sessions was one. They concluded that

---

2. The mode refers to the most frequently occurring number in a series.

this suggests that the client, rather than the therapist, most often determines the length of therapy. Other research on this point is discussed in Hoyt & Talmon (2014).

We do not know whether clients who choose to attend for one session do so by design (ie. it was agreed at the outset that they would attend for one session), or by default (ie. it was agreed that the client would attend for more than one session, but they decided to attend for just one). However, we do know that clients most frequently decide to attend for one session of counselling. The question is why. This brings us to the second rationale for offering SSC to clients.

Most clients who decide to have a single session of counselling are satisfied with the results, given their current circumstances

As noted in the Introduction, recent developments in SSC and walk-in counselling can be traced to the publication of Moshe Talmon's book, *Single-Session Therapy* (1990). With his colleagues Michael Hoyt and Robert Rosenbaum, he did pioneering work on SSC at Kaiser Permanente, a North American integrated managed health care consortium, in the late 1980s. Talmon, an Israeli psychologist, moved in the 1980s from a comfortable private practice in Israel, where most of his clients were in long-term therapy, to working with families and individuals in Kaiser Permanente's public clinic. Over an extended period, he noticed that a large number of his clients only attended one therapy session. He decided to follow up on 200 of these one-session cases, because he wanted to find out what was happening. He discovered to his great surprise that 78% of these clients said that they had got what they wanted from attending therapy and only 10% said that they did not like the therapist or were disappointed with the outcome of therapy. Subsequently, many people have found that between 70% and 80% of clients who have one session of counselling are satisfied with this session, given their current circumstances (see Hoyt & Talmon, 2014).

So, not only do clients in the public and non-profit sectors most commonly attend just one counselling session but they are mostly satisfied with the counselling that they receive. This contrasts with the mindset of most counsellors, who tend to believe that the counselling relationship takes time to develop and that not much can be achieved in a single session. When giving a training workshop on SSC, I ask counsellors how they would feel about standing in front of their colleagues and announcing, 'Most of my clients attend for one session of counselling and choose not to come back.' Most counsellors admit that they would not feel good about doing so – they think it means that their clients have 'dropped out' because they are unhappy with the service they have received. The research evidence shows quite the opposite.

Counsellors are not good at predicting who will attend for one session, and who will attend for more

When a client seeks counselling, their initial contacts with a counselling agency will often be for assessment and history-taking. It is unlikely, therefore, that they will receive counselling at their first point of contact. The purpose of assessment and history-taking is to determine a) whether counselling is the most appropriate form of help for the person, and if so, b) how much counselling is required and of what kind. Such a system works well when an agency has sufficient resources to offer the person what they 'need' and counsellors are accurate in their judgments.[3] However, counsellors are not good at predicting how many sessions a client will attend. This means that time and resources may not be used well in agencies where assessment and history-taking are initial responses to client help-seeking. This is also the case when all clients are offered the same counselling provision once they are deemed suitable for counselling. Thus, everybody may be offered ongoing counselling or, more likely, a block of counselling sessions,[4] despite the fact that, as we have seen, a large number of clients will attend for only one session.

---

3. Who determines what a client needs and the client's role in this judgement is complex and falls outside the scope of this book.

4. Clients are most commonly offered a block of six sessions, but often no clear reason for that number is given.

Given this state of affairs, an alternative way of responding to a client when they seek help is to provide such help from the outset, given that the client is there now because they want help now. They do not particularly want to be assessed or to have their history taken.

Taking these three reasons together, we can say the following. Many clients in the public and non-profit sectors decide to have a single session of counselling and are satisfied with what they get from that session. In response to client help-seeking, counsellors respond by assessing their need for counselling and trying to offer the right kind and right 'dose' of counselling. Research shows that instead they would be far better advised to initiate counselling at the outset, knowing that they have the client in front of them now and they may not see that person again.

In this chapter, I outlined the reasons *why* counsellors should offer SSC to clients. In the next, I will discuss *when* it should be offered.

References

Brown GS, Jones ER (2005). Implementation of a feedback system in a managed care environment: what are patients teaching us? *Journal of Clinical Psychology 61*: 187–198.

Hoyt MF, Talmon MF (2014). What the literature says: an annotated bibliography. In: Hoyt MF, Talmon M (eds). *Capturing the Moment: single session therapy and walk-in services*. Bethel, CT: Crown House Publishing (pp487–516).

Maluccio AN (1979). *Learning from Clients: interpersonal helping as viewed by clients and social workers*. New York, NY: Free Press.

Talmon M (1990). *Single-Session Therapy: maximising the effect of the first (and often only) therapeutic encounter*. San Francisco, CA: Jossey-Bass.

Chapter 3
When should single-session counselling be offered to clients?

Overview and introduction

In this chapter, I will consider the 'when' of SSC. I will discuss the ideas behind the concept of 'help provided at the point of need' – a mode of provision that is in stark contrast to the dominant form, 'help provided at the point of availability'.

I trained as a counsellor in Britain in the mid-1970s. At that time, counselling was in its infancy and the demand for counselling was not strong. Consequently, clients in general did not have to wait for counselling to begin and could be seen for as long as they needed.

As the demand for counselling grew, counselling organisations faced choices as this demand outstripped supply. Some organisations decided to continue to offer clients as much counselling as they needed, with the result that long waiting lists built up. Other organisations decided to cap the number of counselling sessions available to clients and began to offer 'blocks' of counselling.

A block of counselling sessions usually comprises a fixed number of sessions, although it can also refer to a block of time. As I said in Chapter 2, currently the most frequent number of sessions in a block is six, although there is no clear reason for this (it could be five or seven, for example). When the client approaches the end of the block and it seems they need more sessions, in many counselling organisations, the counsellor can apply for this number to be extended. The block of sessions is there to make sure that available counselling resources are equitably distributed, but using these blocks creates waiting lists. In general, the more sessions in a block and the more often such a block is renewed, the longer the waiting list. Moreover, as I mentioned above, the longest waiting lists occur in counselling organisations where no cap is placed on the amount of counselling offered.

Help at the point of need

When a counselling organisation operates a waiting list, they are effectively asking potential clients to wait for help until a 'space' becomes available when that person may be seen. This is known as 'help at the point of availability'. The alternative to 'help at the point of availability' is 'help at the point of need'. Here, as the term makes clear, a person is offered a counselling appointment when they deem it to be necessary. When the demand for counselling exceeds the supply of counsellors, the best way of offering help at the point of need is through SSC. This can either be by appointment or by walk-in. I will discuss both, but first I will outline the ideas that underpin 'help at the point of need.'

Ideas that underpin 'help at the point of need'

If a counselling organisation wishes to offer help at the point of need, it is useful if its counsellors and related staff hold to the following ideas:

1. It is better to respond to client need by providing some help straight away rather than by waiting to provide the best possible help.

Increasingly, particularly with approaches to counselling based on cognitive behaviour therapy, 'treatments' are being offered for certain prescribed 'conditions', such as 'social anxiety disorder', for example. These treatments comprise a set number of sessions and follow explicit, manualised guidelines, often in order. While this is a legitimate approach to therapy, it inevitably leads to lengthening waiting lists for those 'diagnosed' with the relevant condition. So people have a choice: wait for the full treatment or receive help immediately, in a single session, where the agreed intention is to encourage them to derive something therapeutically meaningful from it. SSC practitioners tend to favour the immediate response pathway. In a phrase, 'sooner is better'.

2. Providing immediate help is more important than carrying out a full assessment and/or a case formulation.
When someone seeks counselling, it makes sense from one perspective for the counsellor to begin the process by doing a full assessment of the client's problem(s) and/or a formulation of the 'case' before counselling begins. The downside to this approach is that it tends to lengthen waiting lists and it is predicated on the assumption that clients will remain in counselling long enough to benefit from this approach. As we have already seen, this is not necessarily the case. SSC practitioners consider it more important to offer immediate help.

3. Counselling can be initiated in the absence of a case history.
While it is useful to take a history of the person seeking help, the difficulty is that the counsellor can collect a lot of information that they may well not use. Also, the time the counsellor spends taking the history could be more fruitfully used to offer the person help for their nominated problem. SSC practitioners believe that counselling can be initiated without taking a history of the person. My approach is to ask the person to tell me what they think I need to know about their history in order to help them with their nominated problem. This gives the client the responsibility to point me to the relevant information, rather than me taking the responsibility to spend time finding it.

4. People have the resources to make use of help provided at the point of need.

One of the central ideas on which SSC is based is that people have access to internal strengths and external resources that they can use to help them address their nominated problem. Clients are not functioning well when they come to counselling, and the temptation for counsellors is to focus on this lack of functioning and not on their strengths. Also, there is a temptation to consider aspects of their environment that clients find problematic rather than to focus also on the environmental aspects that they can use to help themselves. In SSC, practitioners ensure that the focus on internal and external resources is kept to the fore.

5. The best way to see if a client will respond well to counselling is by offering them counselling and seeing how they respond.

As noted above, when a client first seeks counselling help, they go through a process of assessment by a representative of the relevant agency. One of the questions this representative asks themself is whether or not the person will respond well to counselling. They may take their views to a case conference meeting, where applications for counselling are considered and prioritised on several criteria, including a client's likely response to counselling. In the same way that counsellors are not good judges of how long clients will remain in counselling (see Chapter 2), they tend not to be good judges about how a client will respond to counselling (Young, 2018). SSC practitioners tend to hold that the best way to discover if a person will respond well to counselling is by offering them counselling and seeing how they respond. Offering someone a single session promptly will help the counsellor see the client's response first-hand. If the person responds well, they may not even require another session; if they do not respond well, another form of help can be suggested, and much time may be saved as a result.

If the best way to see how well a client responds to counselling in general is to offer them a counselling session, the same is true for SSC, as I will discuss in Chapter 5.

6. Counselling can be initiated straight away and risk can be managed if this becomes an issue.

Whenever I run training courses and presentations on SSC, one frequently asked question is 'How can be risk be managed in SSC?' My response is that risk is managed in precisely the same way as it would be in other forms of counselling, but with one difference: the counsellor finds out that the client is at risk sooner in SSC than they would if the client had to wait for a more extended period of counselling to be available. Thus, from one perspective, SSC is safer for clients because help is provided at the point of need, which means they are seen more quickly than when help is provided at the point of availability.

7. The client best determines the length of counselling.

As I discussed in Chapter 2, when a counsellor assesses a client, one point that they keep in mind is how much counselling to offer the person. Some agencies are flexible on this point, and clients will be offered counselling of varying length, depending on the judgement of the person doing the assessment and ratified by a clinical director or clinical team. Other agencies offer clients a block of counselling sessions of similar length, although (as I have pointed out in Chapter 2), the counsellor can apply for more sessions in the block or another block. While it is rare these days, some counselling agencies do offer some or all of their clients ongoing counselling, which presumably continues until the client is ready to end.

Leaving aside the point I have just made, the practices I have outlined here are led by the counsellor, at least at the outset. SSC practitioners take a very different position, and one that is borne out in reality. This is that it is the client who determines the length of counselling, in effect, by choosing to attend sessions, or not to attend. As I have stressed before, all we know for certain in counselling is that the client has chosen to attend the current session (since they are present) and they may or may not decide to attend the next one. SSC rests on this point.

8. When a person does not return for another session, this may well indicate that the person is satisfied with what they have achieved, although it may be the case that they were dissatisfied with the help provided.

An SSC practitioner tends to respond to a client who does not return for a second session of counselling in a different way to a non-SSC practitioner. The latter is likely to assume that this non-return is generally a bad thing, in that the client was dissatisfied with the help they got and they, the counsellor, had not been helpful. Drawing on the research literature (see Hoyt & Talmon, 2014), the SSC practitioner who values offering help provided at the point of need rather than at the point of availability tends to see the client who does not return for a second session in a more positive light. The SSC practitioner knows that counselling lasting a single session is quite common and that the client's non-return is likely to indicate that they were satisfied with the session, given their current circumstances, and does not require further help at that time. However, the SSC practitioner also knows that, in about 25% of cases, the client was not helped or was dissatisfied with the help provided. Thus, the SSC practitioner is realistic but not complacent when a client does not return.

Walk-in counselling

> A specialised form of single-session counselling is known as walk-in counselling. Walk-in counselling is provided in a setting that clearly advertises what it offers. Such counselling enables clients to meet with a mental health professional at their moment of choosing. There is no red tape, no triage, no intake process, no wait list, and no wait. There is no formal assessment, no formal diagnostic process, just one hour of therapy focused on clients' stated wants... Also, with walk-in therapy there are no missed appointments or cancellations, thereby increasing efficiency. (Slive, McElheran & Lawson, 2008: 6)

This definition shows, by implication, the uniqueness of walk-in counselling, in that there is no appointment, whereas in other forms of SSC, an appointment is usually required. So when the client is ready, they 'walk-in' for a counselling session, receive it and tend not to go back.

That said, the person who uses a walk-in counselling service may return as many times as they want, although they usually do not, and it is for people who want a rapid response to a burning issue. The same remarks that I made earlier in this chapter about dealing with clients at risk hold for the way risk is handled in a walk-in service.

The kind of walk-in counselling centre that I am describing here is different from many so-called drop-in centres that exist currently in England. In these centres, people are seen when they 'drop-in', but the response they receive is intended to help them to find the most appropriate service for their problem. They are helped to find their way around the system or are given information that explains more about their problem. What they are not given, by and large, is immediate counselling, designed to help them address their problem there and then, as would be the case if they had walked into a service run on SSC principles.

For more detailed information about walk-in counselling, I recommend that interested readers consult the work of Slive & Bobele (2011, 2014, 2018), who are pioneers in this area of single-session work.

In the next chapter, I will discuss the goals of SSC, from the perspectives of the client and the counsellor.

References

Hoyt MF, Talmon MF (2014). What the literature says: an annotated bibliography. In: Hoyt MF, Talmon M (eds). *Capturing the Moment: single session therapy and walk-in services* . Bethel, CT: Crown House Publishing (pp487–516).

Slive A, Bobele M (2018). The three top reasons why walk-in single sessions make perfect sense. In: Hoyt MF, Bobele M, Slive A, Young J, Talmon M (eds). *Single-Session Therapy by Walk-In or Appointment: administrative, clinical, and supervisory aspects of one-at-a-time services.* New York, NY: Routledge (pp27–39).

Slive A, Bobele M (2014). Walk-in single-session therapy: accessible mental health services. In: Hoyt MF, Talmon M (eds). *Capturing the Moment: single session therapy and walk-in services.* Bethel, CT: Crown House Publishing (pp73–94).

Slive A, Bobele M (eds) (2011). *When One Hour is All You Have: effective therapy for walk-in clients.* Phoenix, AZ: Zeig, Tucker & Theisen.

Slive A, McElheran N, Lawson A (2008). How brief does it get? Walk-in single-session therapy. *Journal of Systemic Therapies 27:* 5–22.

Young J (2018). SST: the misunderstood gift that keeps on giving. In: Hoyt MF, Bobele M, Slive A, Young J, Talmon M (eds). *Single-Session Therapy by Walk-In or Appointment: administrative, clinical, and supervisory aspects of one-at-a-time services.* New York, NY: Routledge (pp40–58).

Chapter 4
The goals of single-session counselling

Overview

Like all forms of counselling, SSC is purposive and both counsellor and client bring a set of goals to the session. Given this, I will discuss their respective goals separately. When considering the client's goals, I will distinguish between session goals and problem-related goals. When considering the counsellor's goals, I will distinguish between outcome goals and process goals.

In this chapter and in the following chapters, I will assume that the client and counsellor have agreed to meet with the expressed intention to help the client deal with whatever the client wants help with in that session, in the knowledge that further help is available.

The client's goals in SSC

The client is likely to have sought counselling because something is going wrong in their life. They have come to counselling because they want to put this right and have entered into a contract for SSC with the counsellor in the hope that they will gain something from that session that will help them along the path to putting things right.

Realistic expectations, SSC and the client's goal

The first thing that I want to stress about the client's goal is that it is vital that the client is realistic about what can be achieved from SSC. On the one hand, it is important that the client holds the idea that they can achieve something meaningful from the session; on the other, they need to recognise that they will probably not achieve 'quantum change' (Miller & C' de Baca, 2001).[1]

While it is vital for the counsellor to ask the client what they want to achieve from the process, it is essential to differentiate between what the client wants to achieve in relation to the problem for which they are seeking help and what they can realistically expect to achieve by the end of the session (ie. between their problem-related goal and their goal for the session). Occasionally, these are the same, and the client achieves more than they hoped they would. However, at the outset, the counsellor needs to help the client focus on their session goal, as the session is occurring in the present and 'now' is the only time the counsellor can be sure that they can be helpful to the person. That being said, it is also important for the counsellor to have an idea about what the client does wish to achieve, so that they can help them see the connection between their goal for the session and their problem-related goal (as shown in Figure 4.1).

---

1. Quantum change points to the phenomenon where a person experiences a sudden personal metamorphosis – as in the case of Scrooge in Charles Dickens' (1843) story, *A Christmas Carol*. Scrooge is portrayed as a cold-hearted miser who despises Christmas and the joy it can bring people. He is transformed overnight by his encounters with three ghostly single-session counsellors (the Ghost of Christmas Present, the Ghost of Christmas Past and the Ghost of Christmas Yet to Come) into a very different person. He becomes more friendly and more generous, as shown by his changed behaviour towards the family of Bob Cratchit, one of his employees, and, in particular, Cratchit's son, Tiny Tim, who would have died had it not been for Scrooge's benevolent intervention.

Figure 4.1: The relationship between the client's problem, their session goal and their problem-related goal

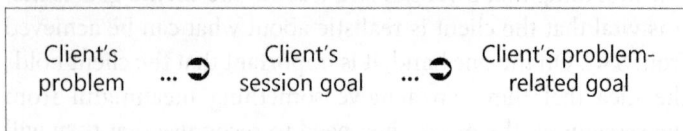

Client's problem	⇢	Client's session goal	⇢	Client's problem-related goal

The client's problem-related goal

When focusing on the client's problem-related goal, the counsellor needs to help them select a target that is clear and realistic. For example, when suggesting a problem-related goal, a client will sometimes talk about the ways they *don't want* to respond to the adversity, rather than how they *do want* to deal with it constructively. Imagine that a client (let's call him Robert) seeks SSC because he has a problem with his manager at work criticising how he does his job. At present, Robert feels hurt and angry (emotional responses) and reacts by getting defensive (behavioural response). When asked for his problem-related goal, Robert says, 'I don't want to feel hurt and angry, and I don't want to get defensive.' While this may sound reasonable, it is problematic because it is based on the implicit idea that a lack of response is healthy. As human beings are not robots, Robert will experience some emotional and behavioural response, given that it is important to him that his work is not criticised.

However, when the client opts for lack of responsiveness as a goal, the counsellor needs to explain that this is neither healthy nor possible and to initiate a conversation about what would constitute a constructive set of emotional and behavioural responses. They need to help the person to construct such a set of responses (eg. 'When my work is criticised, I want to feel disappointed but not hurt or angry, and I want to discuss my manager's feedback in an open way, rather than defensively').

The client's session goal

As can be seen from Figure 4.1, there is a clear connection between the client's goal for the session and the goal that is related to the problem for which they are seeking help. Given this connection, the session goal needs to be something that, if achieved, helps the person to continue to pursue their problem-related goal after the session has been concluded. I call this the 'solution' – if the client implements it, it helps them to address their problem effectively and leads to their achieving their problem-related goal (see Figure 4.2).

Figure 4.2: The relationship between the client's problem, the solution to their problem and their problem-related goal

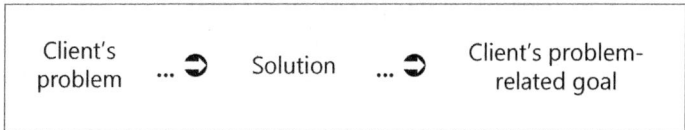

Client's problem	... ⮂	Solution	... ⮂	Client's problem-related goal

Thus, the client is helped to set a session goal that is instrumental in helping them to achieve their problem-related goal. In other words, they are helped to join the counsellor in a search for a solution to their problem. Given this, the client cannot be precise about what the solution will be, since this will be a focus for the session itself. Their session goal, therefore, necessarily will not be precise.

For example, Robert's session goal was: 'To find a way that I can be disappointed about having my work criticised without feeling hurt and angry and to discuss the criticism non-defensively.'

There are several important points to note about the development and use of solutions in SSC, and I will discuss these more fully later. For now, I want to make the following points about solutions:

- Solutions are best regarded in SSC as negotiated by the counsellor and client.

- The counsellor should feel free to offer their ideas to the client about potential solutions, but should do so tentatively. It is unwise to impose potential solutions on a client.

- Given this, the counsellor's ideas may well be a reflection of the counsellor's orientation.

- As will be seen in Chapters 8 and 12, if it is practicable, the client is helped to rehearse the chosen solution in the session and to plan to implement it in their life.

Being listened to and understood

In my experience, clients are, in the main, looking to SSC for solutions that they can implement in order to address their problems effectively. However, sometimes clients are hoping just to be listened to and understood. While the counsellor may explore what *instrumental* value these wishes hold for the client (eg. 'What do you hope to gain by being listened to and understood?'), the client may not be able to articulate what this is, or it may be of secondary importance to its *intrinsic* value. While the search for solutions is understandable for many clients, this is not the case for everyone; the therapeutic power of being given a space to talk and be listened to should never be underestimated and it can make all the difference to some clients, even in a single session.

The counsellor's goals in SSC

The counsellor has several goals in SSC, and these will vary according to the client. Just as with the client's goals, the counsellor's goals can be divided into process goals (those that relate to what the counsellor wants to achieve in the session) and outcome goals (those that are the likely consequence of these process goals and include realistic objectives for the client to achieve from SSC).

The counsellor's outcome goals

The SSC practitioner is optimistic and realistic about what a client can achieve from SSC. In my view, the counsellor's outcome goal for the client can be described in one of the following two ways:

1. To help the client get 'unstuck'.
Very often, when a client seeks help, it is not only because they are in some type of emotional pain but because they are stuck

and are unwittingly doing things that they intend to be helpful to them but that in fact serve to maintain the problem. In this case, the counsellor can seek to help them get 'unstuck' and move on. As shown below, they can best help the client do this by working with them to find a solution to the problem, which here is seen as something that the client can do to help themself move towards their problem-related goal.

2. To help the client take a few steps forward.
Another, similar outcome goal is to help the client take the first few steps towards their problem-related goal, which may help them to travel the rest of the journey without professional assistance. This would involve them using their existing strengths as well as using the solution that they negotiated with the counsellor.

The counsellor's process goals

The counsellor's process goals concern what the counsellor intends to do in the session. The purpose of these activities is to engage the client in SSC and help them to do the work they need to do to achieve their session goals and problem-related goals. The following are the counsellor's major process goals in SSC.

1. To set the parameters for SSC.
Unless the client is engaged in SSC, it is unlikely that much effective work will be done in the session. Consequently, the counsellor needs to ensure that the client understands the nature of SSC and what it realistically can and cannot do. The engagement goes most smoothly when the client has understood all this before they come to the session, and this depends on how successful the agency where the counsellor works has been in disseminating the nature and goals of SSC (see Chapter 9).

Even if the client is clear about what to expect from SSC, it is still worthwhile for the counsellor to make its parameters clear at the outset and to answer any questions the client may have at this point. In clarifying the parameters of SSC, it is vital that the counsellor makes explicit to the client whether or not further help is available and, if so, how the client can access this help.

2. To discover how the client wants the counsellor to best help them.
It is important for the counsellor to discover from the client how they think the counsellor can best help them. This encourages the counsellor to adopt a mode of intervention that is consistent with the client's expectation of how they can best be helped. The exception to this is when, in the counsellor's considered opinion, the client wants to be helped in a way that the counsellor thinks is not helpful to the client. Then the counsellor should feel free to give their reasoning to the client and to indicate how they think they can be more helpful to them.

3. To help the client identify and work with an agreed focus.
In my view, one of the most important process goals the counsellor has in SSC is to help the client to identify a focus and work with that focus throughout the session. This is easiest to achieve when the client nominates a specific problem for which they are seeking help. If the client does not have a specific problem, the counsellor can help them identify one and keep them to it by asking questions such as, 'If you were only able to achieve one thing today that would make coming here worthwhile, what would it be?' The client's response usually helps them both to agree on a focus for the session.

4. To help the client set session and problem-related goals.
In the previous section, I argued that a client is likely to have two goals when coming for SSC: a) a problem-related goal, which is what they would like to achieve concerning their problem, and b) a session goal, most frequently expressed as a solution that helps them to achieve their problem-related goal. Given this, once the counsellor has helped the client to create and maintain a session focus, they then help the client identify a problem-related goal in the first place and a solution-oriented session goal in the second.

5. To help the client see that they have the wherewithal to achieve their goals.
The counsellor may not have time in SSC to help the client address an issue by learning something that is not already in their

repertoire. They do have the time, however, to help the client draw on their established internal strengths and the helping resources that are available to them in their environment. As such, a significant process goal in SSC is for the counsellor to help the client acknowledge and act on the knowledge that they have the wherewithal to achieve their problem-related goal and to implement an agreed solution to their problem.

6. To help the client select a solution to their problem.
Earlier, I made the point that a solution can be most appropriately seen as lying between the client's identified problem or issue and the goal that they have nominated concerning that problem or issue (see Figure 4.2). The counsellor may have a clear idea of what the best solution is for that client, and this may be based on whatever therapeutic orientation the counsellor favours. However, in SSC, the counsellor needs to encourage the client to be an active participant in the search for the best solution for them to use at this particular moment in their life. This may involve the counsellor discovering any solutions the client has tried in the past and the outcomes of these attempts to help themself. As will be discussed in Chapters 8 and 12, the counsellor encourages the client to take the lead in the search for potential solutions but they should also feel free to *invite* the client to say whether or not they are interested in their (the counsellor's)thoughts on the matter.

Finally, the search for a solution is not focused on the best possible solution to the client's problem but on the solution that the client is most likely to use, given their current circumstances.

7. To give the client the experience of the solution in the session, if possible.
It is only when a client tries out the solution that they can tell whether or not it will help them and whether or not they will be able to implement it after the session has finished. If, having tried it, the client thinks a different solution is indicated, then they and the counsellor will explore why the initially selected solution has not worked, which will help them select one that will be more effective.

8. To help the client develop an action plan.
Once the counsellor and client have agreed on a solution, then the counsellor helps the client to devise a plan to implement the solution going forward.

9. To end the session well and clarify with the client how to access future help.
This is a vital process goal for the counsellor – to bring the session to a good conclusion, having given the client an opportunity to raise any last-minute issues and clarified with the client if, when and how they can access more help if needed.

In the next chapter, I will discuss who SSC is intended for.

References

Dickens C (1843). *A Christmas Carol in Prose: being a ghost story of Christmas*. London: Chapman & Hall.

Miller WR, C' de Baca J (2001). *Quantum Change: when epiphanies and sudden insights transform ordinary lives*. New York, NY: Guilford.

Chapter 5
Who is single-session counselling for?

Overview

At first sight, it is perfectly reasonable for counsellors to ask the question, 'Who is single-session counselling for?' There are four ways of addressing the issues that are raised by this question, and I will consider each in this chapter. They are to:

- fully engage with the question
- consider what walk-in services tell us about the question
- let clients choose
- embed SSC with other modes of counselling delivery.

Fully engage with the question

When one fully engages with the question of who SSC is for, it leads one to consider the indications and contraindications for it. When I first developed my approach to single-session work that I use in private practice, which I call single-session integrated cognitive behaviour counselling (SSI-CBT), I outlined several indications and contraindications for it (Dryden, 2017). Extrapolating from these to SSC, this way of approaching the question reveals the following.

Indications for SSC

Non-clinical problems

In general, people with non-clinical problems[1] are the most suited for SSC. These include:

- people with common, non-clinical emotional problems of living (problematic forms of anxiety, non-clinical depression, guilt, shame, anger, hurt, jealousy and envy)

- people with relationship issues at home and at work

- people with everyday problems of self-discipline

- people who are ready to take care of business now and whose problem is non-clinical but suitable for a single-session approach

- people who are stuck and need some help to get unstuck and move on

- people with clinical problems, but who are ready to tackle a non-clinical problem

- people with life dilemmas and quandaries

- people who need to make an important imminent decision

- people who are finding it difficult to adjust to life in some way

- people with meta-emotional problems (emotional problems about emotional problems)

- people in need of prompt and focused crisis management.

Clinical problems

While most would argue that clinical problems require more than a single session, there are examples in the literature where

1. By non-clinical problems, I mean where the person experiences problems of living in the mild to moderate range of distress. These problems are acute rather than chronic. By clinical problems, I mean where the person experiences psychological problems in the severe range of distress. These problems tend to be chronic rather than acute.

such problems can be addressed successfully in one session. Simple phobias can be addressed effectively in an intensive single session lasting up to three hours (Davis III, Ollendick & Öst, 2012) and panic disorder in a single session (Reinecke et al, 2013). Both approaches involve actual exposure to the threat and clients are those who are ready to take care of business and ready to do what they need to do to address these problems effectively.

Coaching

So far, I have discussed the indications of SSC for clients who have problems that they want help for, whether these are non-clinical or clinical in nature. SSC can also be used with people seeking help with getting more out of themselves, their work, their relationships and their life in general. These people are doing OK in the various aspects of their lives, and/or in their lives in general, but have the sense that they are not fulfilling their potential. The focus of this work is usually referred to as 'coaching', whether this label is used to describe the work formally or informally. While coaching is usually a longer-term process, it can be used in a single session format. This is the case when the person wants a session with a coach to kickstart a process that they want to do on their own or they have a specific objective that they think they can achieve at the end of a single, focused session (Dryden, 2019).

Prevention

There are occasions when people are given a warning by a health professional – for example, that they need to take action to prevent the development of a problem – and seek prophylactic help. Given this, much can be achieved with SSC.

Psychoeducation

Psychoeducation involves the provision of information and experiences designed to help a person learn more about a psychological problem, process or treatment (also see Lukens & McFarlane, 2004). A single session where psychoeducation is the focus might be suitable where:

- people are open to counselling, but want to try it first before committing themselves
- people are seeking advice on how counselling would tackle their problem
- people are reluctant about seeking counselling and are only prepared to commit to one session
- counselling trainees want to find out what it is like to have counselling from a different perspective.

Other contexts

Other situations where SSC might be indicated include:

- clients in counselling who are seeking a second opinion (or their counsellors are)
- clients in ongoing counselling who want brief help with a problem with which their counsellor cannot or will not help them
- people who are only in the area for a short period and need some help locally.

SSC can also be used when people volunteer for a demonstration session before an audience or volunteer for a videotaped demonstration session

Contraindications for SSC

There are several conditions where SSC may not be appropriate. They include:

- people who find it challenging to connect with or trust a counsellor quickly
- people who request ongoing counselling
- people who do not want counselling of any description
- people who need ongoing counselling
- people who have vague complaints and cannot be specific
- people who are likely to feel abandoned by the counsellor.

However, the above analysis is based on a number of points:

1. It is desirable to determine who is suitable and unsuitable for a single session before that session takes place.

2. It is possible to determine who is suitable and unsuitable for a single session before that session takes place.

3. Such judgements have a high degree of validity.

While it may be desirable to determine who is suitable and unsuitable for SSC, it may not be possible to do so in a timely fashion. It was when I realised that I was spending a single session deciding if someone was suitable for single-session counselling that I abandoned the quest for SSC suitability and unsuitability criteria. Today, I am sceptical that the judgements that I and others have made about such criteria have a high degree of validity. The experiences of those who work in walk-in centres (see below) have shown that sometimes clients who might be expected to benefit from SSC do not do so and sometimes clients who might be expected not to benefit from SSC actually do so.

The walk-in argument

Walk-in counselling is single-session counselling that occurs when a client walks into a centre without an appointment and is offered counselling straight away. As I have already pointed out, this is counselling provided at the point of need rather at the point of availability. I distinguish between walk-in centres, where counselling is provided from the first moment, and drop-in centres, where clients are seen quite quickly and the thrust of the help is to signpost them to different forms of help so they can choose the right type for them. Even if counselling is indicated as the most appropriate form of help for the person, they are unlikely to be offered it at that point and will be referred to an agency providing counselling.

At a walk-in centre, the client turns up and is offered help immediately. They do not go through a screening process first. It may be that counselling is not appropriate for them, but this is decided between the counsellor and the client, based on experience, not conjecture. Often the best way to discover if counselling is appropriate for a person is to engage them in counselling.

Let the client choose

As noted earlier, SSC is a mode of delivering counselling services that is best offered alongside other modes of counselling delivery. When this happens, a client is presented with a choice about what counselling mode they deem most suitable. When the client thinks that they can be best helped by SSC, they are effectively referring themself to SSC. As SSC begins from the first moment, it will soon become clear whether or not the client will benefit from the session. If not, then the counsellor and client can discuss this openly and decide together what to do. This will usually result in the client accessing a different mode of counselling delivery.

The embedded approach

The final approach is provided by Jeff Young, whose response to the question about suitability and unsuitability for SSC (or SST, as he calls it) is as follows:

> We believe the best response to this question is to avoid having to answer it by embedding SST in the service system so that clients can return if they want to. Embedding SST into the service system so that all services the organization normally provides are available following an initial session, conducted as if it may be the last, allows the practitioner and the organization to avoid the 'difficult if not impossible' decision of who is suitable and who is not suitable for a 'one-off' session. (Young, 2018: 48-49)

In the next chapter, I will discuss SSC's foundational principles.

References

Davis III TE, Ollendick TH, Öst L-G (eds) (2012). *Intensive One-Session Treatment of Specific Phobias.* New York, NY: Springer.

Dryden W (2019). *Single-Session Coaching and One-At-A-Time Coaching: distinctive features.* Abingdon: Routledge.

Dryden W (2017). *Single-Session Integrated CBT (SSI-CBT): distinctive features.* Abingdon: Routledge.

Lukens EP, McFarlane WR (2004). Psychoeducation as evidence practice: considerations for practice, research and policy. *Brief Treatment and Crisis Intervention 4*: 205–225.

Reinecke A, Waldenmaier L, Cooper MJ, Harmer CJ (2013). Changes in automatic threat processing precede and predict clinical changes with exposure-based cognitive-behavior therapy for panic disorder. *Biological Psychiatry 73*: 1064-1070.

Young J (2018). SST: the misunderstood gift that keeps on giving. In: Hoyt MF, Bobele M, Slive A, Young J, Talmon J, Talmon M (eds). *Single-Session Therapy by Walk-In or Appointment: administrative, clinical, and supervisory aspects of one-at-a-time services .* New York, NY: Routledge (pp40–58).

Chapter 6
The principles of single-session counselling

Overview

In this chapter, I will outline and discuss several important principles on which SSC rests. These are:

- the power of now
- even a brief encounter can be therapeutic
- the expandable nature of counselling length
- the importance of client readiness and capitalising on this readiness
- the strengths-based emphasis of SSC
- factors external to counselling may be at least as important as those internal to the client
- reciprocity in openness and feedback.

The power of now

One of the most important principles on which SSC rests is 'the power of now' (Tolle, 2005). The SSC practitioner often does not know with any degree of certainty that the client in front of them will return for a second session, even when this has been planned. The only certainty the counsellor has is that they have the client in front of them, to work with 'now', so why not do as much as possible in the time that the client is with them?

So many other modes of counselling delivery are based on the idea of help happening in the future. This means that activities in the 'now' tend to be undertaken with the future in mind. For example, in future-oriented help, clients are assessed 'now' for help that will be offered in the future. While this may seem sensible, the client may not come back for the future help. Ironically, they may have been satisfied with the help provided when they were being assessed for future-oriented help (Hoyt & Talmon, 2014). I use an image to remind me of the power of now (see Figure 6.1) and have a similar physical 'now' clock in my office.

Figure 6.1: The 'now' clock

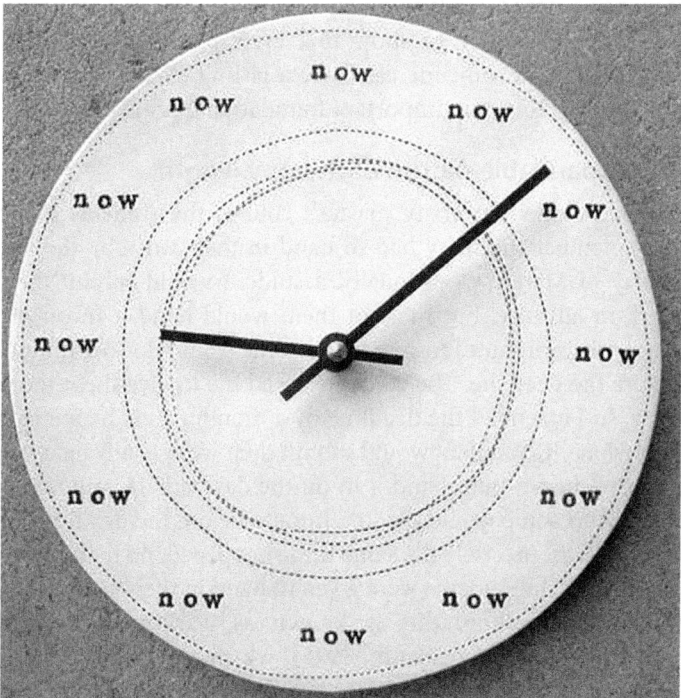

Even a brief encounter can be therapeutic

Many years ago, when I was in my late teens, I was listening on the radio to an interview with Michael Bentine (1922–1996), one of the original Goons and the creator of the popular (at the time) children's TV programme 'Potty Time'. In the course of the hour-long interview, Bentine discussed very briefly his experiences of having a stammer and what he found helpful in dealing with his speech impediment. One technique he found helpful was developing and practising the attitude, 'If I stammer, I stammer. Too bad.'

I have a lifelong stammer, which was much worse then than it is now. Also, I was anxious about stammering then, which I am not now. I remember being very impressed with Bentine's self-helping attitude and resolved to implement this myself. I did try it, and it helped me greatly to calm down about the prospect of stammering, which in turn encouraged me to speak up when before I had kept quiet.

I tell this story to show that even a very brief, virtual encounter with someone can have a lasting effect. Applied to counselling, this is an important foundational principle of SSC.

The expandable nature of therapy length

When I ran a university master's course, the students knew in September that they had to hand in their work by the last Friday in March. Occasionally, a student would submit their work in advance, but most of them would hand it in on the day, with 15 minutes to spare, and some would do so a minute before the deadline. The students asked me to give them more time, so I extended the deadline by a month. What happened? Occasionally, a student would submit their work in advance, but most of them would hand it in on the day with 15 minutes to spare, and some would do so a minute before the deadline. In other words, precisely the same thing happened, no matter how much time the students were given to hand in their work.

In counselling, this is known as 'Parkinson's law in psychotherapy' (Appelbaum, 1975), which states that therapy expands and contracts to fill the time allocated to it. As Moshe

Talmon (1993: 135), one of the developers of modern SSC, has put it:

> Therapy takes exactly the length of time allocated for it. When the therapist and client expect change to happen now, it often does.

The importance of client readiness and capitalising on this readiness

Readiness to change is an important foundational principle of SSC. Much can be achieved if the client is ready and the counsellor can capitalise on their readiness. When the client is ready to change, they are most open to what the therapist has to offer. So, when a person seeks counselling and is ready to change, it is important for the counsellor to offer them help there and then. So many counsellors respond to client readiness to change by assessing the person's suitability for counselling, taking a case history or carrying out a case formulation of their problems, rather than helping them at the outset. There is nothing wrong with these activities of themselves, but they all serve to take the client away from what they want – to receive help at the very point when they are ready to use it.

Let me give an example of this. Many years ago, a woman, whom I shall call 'Vera', sought help from Albert Ellis for her elevator (lift) phobia. For financial reasons, she joined one of his groups but, despite finding the group supportive, she had made minimal progress after being in it for about a year. At that point, Vera made another individual appointment to see Albert Ellis. She rushed into his office late on a Friday afternoon and pleaded with him: 'Dr Ellis, you have to help me get over my phobia by Monday morning!' She explained that her work office had always been on the fifth floor of a skyscraper but, over the coming weekend, they were moving to the 105th floor of the same building. 'I can just about walk up and down five floors of stairs, but there is no way I can walk up and down 105 floors. I need my job, Dr Ellis, you have to help me!' she told him. Albert Ellis helped her by reminding her that she knew what she needed to do – to go up and down elevators until she no longer felt anxious about doing so. This is what she did. She spent that evening, all day Saturday and up to Sunday afternoon riding on elevators until she was no longer anxious.

In my view, there are four components of client readiness to change:

1. Knowing what to do to change.

2. Having a committed reason to change.

3. Taking appropriate action.

4. Being prepared to tolerate any costs involved.

From this analysis, it is clear why Vera did not benefit from therapy in the first instance. She knew what to do, but she did not have a committed reason to change. Therefore she did not take the appropriate action and she did not experience any costs from not changing. In the second instance, she again knew what to do, but this time she had a clear reason to take action, and she was prepared to tolerate the significant discomfort of doing so.

The case of Vera shows the importance of client readiness, the components of such readiness and the willingness of the counsellor to capitalise on that readiness.

Using the 'stages of change' model

One model that is particularly useful when considering the concept of readiness to change in SSC is that of the 'stages of change'. Originally designed for therapeutic work with people with substance abuse problems, this model has been applied more broadly in the field of counselling. There are a number of versions of the model. The one I hold in mind when practising SSC outlines six stages of change:

1. Pre-contemplation. When a person is in the pre-contemplation phase of change, they do not acknowledge that they have a problem. Others may think that they have a problem, but they do not.

2. Contemplation. Here, the person is beginning to think that they may have a problem, but they are still in two minds about it.

3. Preparation. Here, the person has decided that they do have a problem and is researching how to address it.

4. Action. Here, the person has decided on a course of action and is implementing it.

5. Maintenance. In this stage, the person has taken action and achieved their goal, but now needs to maintain what they have achieved. During this stage, the person identifies and deals productively with lapses.

6. Relapse. In this stage, the person has failed to deal effectively with lapses and has relapsed and gone 'back to square one' in the change process.

I use this model within the SSC framework to determine which stage of change a client is in when they seek help, and respond accordingly. I am guided by the notion that the minimum goal I set myself is to help the person move from one stage to another. I do not assume that, because they are seeking help, they are in the preparation, action or maintenance stage of change. If it turns out that they are in the pre-contemplation stage of change, my own approach is to underscore the point that they do not have to stay in the session if they do not want to. I will outline how I see my role and invite them to come back to see me if they want to explore the possibility that they may have a problem (ie. they are in the contemplation stage) or they have decided that they have a problem and want to do something about it. Allowing the person the right not to have a problem minimises resistance and may lead them to stand back and reconsider their decision on this point.

The strengths-based emphasis of SSC

People who come to therapy frequently focus on their perceived weaknesses and deficits, as these crystallise into the problem for which they are seeking help. In SSC, the counsellor takes these factors seriously but also encourages the client to identify their own strengths that they can draw on as they and their counsellor work to address the problem effectively. Sometimes, particularly when they are quite demoralised, the client claims that they do not have any such strengths. In response, the counsellor can ask questions such as:

- 'If you were at a job interview and were asked what strengths you have that you could use while addressing your problem, what would you say?'

- 'What would a very good friend who knows you exceptionally well say are your strengths that could be particularly useful in addressing your problem?' (Dryden, 2019).

It may be helpful for the counsellor to give some examples of strengths to kick-start the process if the client struggles with the concept.

Factors external to counselling may be at least as important as those internal to the client

Strengths may be seen as factors internal to the client that, when used, could facilitate the client in achieving their goal. Factors external to the client can sometimes be just as important to the change process. For example, a client (I will call him Lee), came to see me in person for SSC (Dryden, 2017) following a pre-session telephone contact. The night before he came to see me, he met up with a group of his male friends who he had not seen for a while. He told them why he was in town – he was to see a counsellor for difficulties he was experiencing following the death of his mother. His friends empathised and most shared that they had faced similar challenges. Lee found this a great comfort to him and allowed himself to feel the grief he had hitherto seen as a weakness. When I saw him the next day, he had effectively achieved what he wanted from the session without having had the session.

Thus, SSC practitioners give as much weight to these external resources as potential change agents as they do to the client's internal factors.

Reciprocity in openness and feedback

This is the final principle on which SSC rests, and it relates both to the counsellor and the client.

Counsellor openness and feedback

The counsellor seeks to be open about what they can and cannot do in SSC. They are also open about the solutions they think may be helpful to the client. A vivid example of this occurs in single-session family counselling. In family therapy, there is a tradition that, when one or two therapists work with a family, their work is observed live by a group of colleague therapists, from outside the room. Sometime during the session, the therapists who are working directly with family will take a break, leave the room and consult with the team of observing therapists. Together, the entire group will suggest a number of interventions to address the family's issues. The main point to bear in mind here is that this discussion is carried out in the *absence* of the family. In single-session family counselling, instead of leaving the therapy room to join the observing team at the break, the working therapists stay with the family and are joined by the observing team. The ensuing open discussion occurs in the *presence* of the family members, who are encouraged to join the discussion and give feedback on the potential usefulness of the suggested interventions.

Client openness and feedback

The client is encouraged to be open throughout the session about the following issues:

- the problem they want to prioritise for the session
- how they think the counsellor can best help them
- how they have addressed the problem in the past and the effect of their attempts

- what they would like to achieve from the session
- their ideas of potential solutions to the problem
- what they think of the counsellor's solution suggestions
- what they will take away from the session.

At follow-up, they are encouraged to give honest feedback on what they think about the service they have received. The counsellor uses this feedback to modify their future practice.

In the next chapter, I will discuss the conditions in which SSC thrives and the conditions in which it withers.

References

Appelbaum SA (1975). Parkinson's law in psychotherapy. *International Journal of Psychoanalytic Psychotherapy* 4: 426–436.

Dryden W (2019). *Single-Session Therapy: 100 key points and techniques.* Abingdon: Routledge.

Dryden W (2017). *Single-Session Integrated CBT (SSI-CBT): distinctive features.* Abingdon: Routledge.

Hoyt MF, Talmon MF (2014). What the literature says: an annotated bibliography. In: Hoyt MF, Talmon M (eds). *Capturing the Moment: single session therapy and walk-in services.* Bethel, CT: Crown House Publishing (pp487–516).

Talmon M (1993). *Single-Session Solutions: a guide to practical, effective and affordable therapy.* New York, NY: Addison-Wesley.

Tolle E (2005). *The Power of Now: a guide to spiritual enlightenment.* London: Hodder & Stoughton.

Chapter 7
When does single-session counselling thrive and when does it wither?

Overview

In this chapter, I will invite you to think of SSC as a plant. Different plants need different conditions to thrive. Conditions that will lead one plant to thrive may lead a different plant to wither and die. So here I will consider which conditions encourage SSC to thrive and which result in it withering.

Favourable conditions for SSC

In this opening section of the chapter, I will discuss eight favourable conditions for SSC. The more these conditions are present, the more SSC will thrive.

Shared intentionality

In Chapter 1, I defined SSC as 'a purposeful endeavour where the counsellor and client meet with the intention that one session may be sufficient, but with the understanding that more sessions may be available'. Thus, 'intentionality' is a favourable condition for SSC, and what is important to avoid is a situation where the counsellor intends to work within an SSC framework but the client expects longer, ongoing counselling. This shared intentionality is made concrete when the client gives their informed consent to move forward with the session. Similarly, SSC will not thrive when the client is looking for help within a single-session framework and the counsellor is offering longer-term work.

Shared realistic expectations

Both counsellor and client may approach the session with the intention of helping the client in a single session, knowing that more help is available. However, the two may not share realistic expectations about SSC. Thus, it is the counsellor's responsibility to raise the issue of expectations with the client and, if necessary, help them to be more realistic in what to expect before embarking on the process. I assume here that the SSC practitioner holds realistic expectations themself.

Help is provided quickly when help is sought

It makes little sense for a client to come to SSC with realistic expectations and with the intention of using that session to get what they want from counselling and move on if they have to wait for an appointment. This compromises the power of SSC. SSC depends in large part on the power of 'now' (see Chapter 6), and if the client cannot access help when they are ready to use it, they may no longer be ready when it is offered to them at a later – sometimes much later – date.

The time between help-seeking and the counselling session is used well

SSC can occur by walk-in or by appointment. But even when the person comes to a walk-in clinic for a single session of counselling, there may be a short wait before the person can be seen by a counsellor. While they wait, they may be asked to complete a short form designed to help them get the most from the session. The same is true if someone makes an appointment for SSC.

If a person makes an appointment to see a counsellor for SSC, usually they will be sent literature about the practices of the counselling agency with whom they are making the appointment, or of the counsellor if the work is to take place in private practice. Alternatively, or in addition, the client may be sent a pre-counselling form designed to help them get the most from the session. If they do not want to complete it in advance, they may be asked to come in a half an hour before their appointment to do so.

This productive use of time is a feature of effective SSC. Practitioners and agencies need to think about how they can encourage clients to use time effectively between help-seeking and the session. However, here, as elsewhere, client choice should be respected. Clients should be invited to use such time effectively, not be pressured to do so.

Clarity

Clarity throughout SSC facilitates communication between counsellor and client and helps the client get the most out of the process. The following are several areas where clarity is particularly helpful in SSC:

- SSC is explained clearly on the agency's or counsellor's website so the client is able to decide whether or not to seek SSC and what to expect.

- When they first meet face to face, the counsellor is clear about what SSC can and cannot offer the client.

- The counsellor makes it clear to the client if and what help is available after the session and how they can access it.

- Throughout SSC, the counsellor speaks clearly and at a speed that helps the client process the information.

- The counsellor ensures that the client understands any substantive points or concepts they have used during SSC. This is best done by inviting the client to put into their own words their understanding of the counsellor's communication and for the counsellor to correct any misunderstandings this reveals.

Effective goal-setting

In Chapter 4, I discussed the client's and the counsellor's goals in SSC. From the perspective of creating favourable conditions for SSC, it is important that the client sets a meaningful goal for the session – one that can be achieved by the application of an agreed solution. Counsellor and client agreement on the client's goal is important in that it strengthens the working alliance between the two, and a strong working alliance is associated with a good client outcome in SSC (Simon et al, 2012).

Organisational, training and administrative support are provided

It is important that SSC operates in an environment that can support it.

a) Organisational support: interpersonal. From an organisational perspective, favourable conditions are both interpersonal and physical. For SSC to thrive in an organisation, all stakeholders need to see its value and support it. Relevant stakeholders include directors of the organisation, managers, client representatives and counsellors. As I will discuss more fully in Chapter 15, counsellors in particular are challenged by some of the principles and practices of SSC. It is important that such counsellors have an opportunity to voice their concerns about SSC and to engage in an open, respectful discussion with those who have a positive attitude towards it. It is important to realise that SSC is not for all counsellors, just as it won't suit all clients, and only counsellors who are positively inclined towards SSC should practise it. Counsellors should not be pressurised into practising SSC when they do not wish to do so.

b) Organisational support: physical. SSC may receive interpersonal support in a counselling agency but still not thrive because it is not given enough physical support. Thus, SSC needs to be practised in an agency where there are enough counselling rooms and an appropriate waiting area. If SSC is being provided by walk-in, then ideally the service needs to be accessible but discreet.

c) **Training support.** As we have seen, the most frequent number of sessions that clients have in public and non-profit counselling agencies is one. However, counsellors are, in general, not trained in SSC as part of their foundation training. If an organisation wants SSC to thrive in the longer term, then it needs to provide training in SSC for its counsellors.

d) **Administrative support.** As we have seen, SSC thrives in a setting where help is provided quickly at the point of need. The role of administrators, therefore, is crucial, to enable this to happen as smoothly as possible. They need to understand SSC and support its aims. Involving key administrative staff in training events is therefore recommended.

The counsellor brings their expertise to the session without assuming the role of expert

Because SSC encourages clients to draw on their own strengths in addressing the issues for which they are seeking help, SSC practitioners are very wary of being perceived as experts by their clients. Their concern is that, if clients perceive them as experts, they will rely on them, and not on themselves, for generating solutions to their problems. Consequently, I believe, counsellors are reluctant to share their expertise with their clients.

I think this is a mistake. If clients are invited to bring their strengths to the SSC process, surely counsellors can bring their expertise, while simultaneously promoting client autonomy. Thus, after eliciting the client's view about the nature of their problem and the factors that account for it, the counsellor can ask the client if they are interested in their (the counsellor's) views on this issue. Once the client indicates such an interest, the counsellor can offer their view and initiate a discussion, the purpose of which is to arrive at a shared perspective that can be used by both going forward.

Unfavourable conditions for SSC

The conditions under which SSC will wither are revealed simply by reversing the points above. However, I do wish to highlight some common practices in counselling organisations that would make the establishment and maintenance of SSC problematic.

Help is provided when it is available

Most counselling agencies operate a service based on help being provided to people when it becomes available, rather than when it is needed by the person. From one perspective, this is understandable in such a situation: if the agency thinks it is important to provide ongoing counselling, unless they have a lot of counsellors to staff such a service, the demand for the services will inevitably exceed the resources they have to meet it. Under these conditions, SSC would not thrive.

Blocks of sessions are offered

One approach that counselling agencies have adopted to respond to growing waiting lists, where demand outstrips supply, is to limit the number of counselling sessions offered to clients. Blocks of limited numbers of counselling sessions are offered to all people seeking help. While the use of blocks reduces the time that people have to wait for an appointment, they are still associated with waiting lists. All things being equal, the more sessions in a 'block', the longer the waiting list and, as we have seen, SSC does not thrive in an environment where people have to wait for help.

The use of blocks of counselling also runs counter to how many people in public and non-profit counselling agencies use counselling. As we have seen, the most frequent number of counselling sessions that people have is one, followed by two, three and so on (Hoyt & Talmon, 2014). This suggest that blocks of sessions should not be routinely offered to clients, since clients tend not to stay for the full number of sessions. I am not saying that blocks of sessions should not be offered to clients. Rather, I am saying that they should be offered when there is a good therapeutic reason to do so. The most common number of sessions in a block tends to be six, in my experience. I haven't yet been given a good clinical reason for the choice of six sessions. I am told that it is six because it has always been six.

This is not acceptable in this day and age, where such decisions need to be based on research evidence.

Help is provided after certain conditions have been met

Counselling agencies that offer help at the point of availability do not offer help immediately because people in authority tend to believe that certain clinical activities need to occur first. The purpose of these activities is to ensure that clients get the right type of help. Again, I am not decrying such practices *per se.* However, I am saying that they are inimical to the development and maintenance of SSC.

These clinical practices tend to be:

a) A full assessment. Here, the client is fully assessed in all relevant areas of their life before counselling begins. A full case history is undertaken and a case formulation developed (see below). This can take several sessions and significantly delays the start of counselling, placing it at variance with the ethos of SSC, with its emphasis on help provided at the point of need.

b) Case formulation. A case formulation has been defined as:

> ... the clinician's collective understanding of the client's problems as viewed through a particular theoretical orientation; as defined by the biological, psychological, and social contexts of the client; and as supported by a body of research and practice that links a set of co-occurring symptoms to a diagnosis and, ultimately, a treatment plan. A strong case conceptualization is guided by the utilization of a theoretical orientation that provides a framework for the clinician from which to condense and synthesize multiple pieces of information into a coherent and well-developed narrative. This narrative aims to identify not only the precipitating cause(s) of the client's problems but also the forces at work, both internal and external to the client, that serve to maintain the problems.
> (John & Segal, 2015)

I want to stress here that there is nothing wrong with developing a case formulation with a client when that person has several interlocking problems and there is a high degree of probability that they will engage with and remain in ongoing counselling so the treatment suggested by the case formulation can be undertaken. However, from the perspective of SSC, with its focus on the problem that the client most wants help with, such a case formulation is not necessary and, because it takes quite a while to develop, prevents help being provided straight away.

c) **Case history.** A case history in counselling usually involves the counsellor asking the client a series of questions designed to help them understand the psychological development of the person, particularly where this is relevant but not limited to their presenting concerns. The counsellor usually gains a great deal of information about the client, much of which may not be used during the actual counselling. As such, taking a case history is usually detrimental to SSC. An alternative approach in SSC is to ask the client a question such as, 'Is there anything I need to know about you that is essential for me to know as we address your problem?' This hands to the client the responsibility for informing the counsellor of any crucial information. When the counsellor assumes this responsibility, they can end up taking a case history.

There is a long gap between help being sought and help being provided

For whatever reason, when there is a long gap between help being sought and help being offered, the consequence may be that, when help is eventually provided, the client may not be in the same state of readiness to address their problem as they were when they first sought help. Consequently, if SSC is offered under these circumstances, its therapeutic potency would be diminished.

The time between the client's initial contact and help being provided is not used or not used well

I hope it is clear by now that SSC thrives when the time available is used well by both counsellor and client. What generally happens in counselling agencies offering help at the point of availability is that, when a person makes initial contact, they are informed of the length of the waiting list and offered or directed to online or self-help resources that may be broadly relevant to their concern but unlikely to be tailored to their situation. Contrast this with what I outlined earlier, in the section 'The time between help-seeking and the counselling session is used well'. Here the waiting period between the person's initial contact and the session is short and, during the time between the two, the person is helped to prepare for and to get the most from the session.

There is a lack of organisational, training and/or administrative support

When there is lack of organisational, training and/or administrative support, even the most enthusiastic efforts of SSC advocates will eventually fail. For example, in one university counselling service in England, a senior counsellor who opposed SSC was eventually able to get the service closed down, even though it ran successfully for three years. The junior staff member originally tasked with setting up the SSC service was not given a full reason for its closure and was not even present when the decision was taken.

In the next chapter, I get down to the nitty-gritty of what constitutes good and bad practice in SSC.

References

Hoyt MF, Talmon MF (2014). What the literature says: an annotated bibliography. In: Hoyt MF, Talmon M (eds). *Capturing the Moment: single session therapy and walk-in services*. Bethel, CT: Crown House Publishing (pp487–516).

John S, Segal DL (2015). Case conceptualization. In: Cautin RL, Lilienfeld SO (eds). *The Encyclopedia of Clinical Psychology*. [Online.] Chichester: John Wiley & Sons. http://onlinelibrary.wiley.com/doi/10.1002/9781118625392.wbecp106/abstract (accessed July 2019).

Simon GE, Imel ZE, Ludman EJ, Steinfeld BJ (2012). Is dropout after a first psychotherapy visit always a bad outcome? *Psychiatric Services 63*(7): 705–707.

Chapter 8
Good practice and bad practice in single-session counselling

Overview

In this chapter, I go to the heart of SSC, which is its practice. Having made the point that counsellors from any therapeutic orientation can practise SSC, I will discuss 'good' and 'bad' practice in this mode of counselling deivery. By good practice, I mean elements of SSC practice that counsellors should try to implement. By bad practice, I mean elements of its practice that counsellors should try to avoid. However, given the flexible nature of SSC practice, there will be exceptions to these principles.

Good practice in SSC

What follows is a list of 'transtherapeutic'[1] interventions that are associated with good practice in SSC. I will briefly discuss each one.

---

1. By 'transtherapeutic', I mean ways of practising SSC that are common across therapeutic orientations.

Develop the working alliance at the outset and maintain it throughout

It has been shown that, when clients derive benefit from SSC, they have a good working alliance with their counsellors. Conversely, when they do not derive benefit, a good working alliance has not been developed (Simon et al, 2012). In my reformulation of Bordin's (1979) tripartite model of the working alliance, I argued that there are four domains of this alliance: bonds, goals, views and tasks (Dryden, 2011). A good alliance in SSC is characterised by a well-bonded relationship (*bonds*), with both parties in agreement on the *goals* of the session. The counsellor and the client negotiate shared *views* about the factors that have led to the problem, those that maintain the problem and those that may lead to the resolution of the problem. Finally, both parties agree on the *tasks* that they need to carry out in order that the client achieves their goals. Once the alliance has been established, both counsellor and client need to work to maintain it.

Be clear with the client concerning the purpose of the session and what can and cannot be achieved

In Chapter 4, I referred to the Dickens character, Scrooge, who went to bed on Christmas Eve a cranky, mean-spirited old man and, after being visited by the Ghosts of Christmas Past, Christmas Present and Christmas Yet to Come, woke up on Christmas Day a radically changed man. It is important for the counsellor to make clear that this is not the purpose of SSC. Rather, the counsellor is there to help the client take a meaningful step towards change.

Ask the client how they think they can best be helped

The SSC practitioner does not possess magical insight into the best helping stance to take towards the client. Rather, they should ask the client directly, and if the client is not clear, the counsellor should give them a few different examples to stimulate their thinking. The counsellor should be guided by the client but should not offer what the client suggests if they deem it not to be constructive. In this case, they should give their reasons for not doing so and negotiate a different form of helping instead.

Ask what the client wants to achieve from the session, rather than from therapy

Even though the client probably has some idea of what they want from therapy, asking them what they want to achieve from the session concentrates their mind and helps them to focus on the 'now'. By doing so, the counsellor is communicating to the client that they can derive benefit from the session.

Ask what the client is prepared to sacrifice to achieve their goal

Once the client has nominated a goal, they can be asked what they are prepared to sacrifice in order to achieve it. For example, if the client's nominated problem is anxiety and they want to address it effectively, they will need to tolerate discomfort in order to do so.

Be focused and encourage the client to stay focused

Knowing what the client wants to get from the session helps the counsellor to establish a shared focus with the client. Once the focus is created, it is the counsellor's primary responsibility to help them both to stay focused. This may involve the counsellor interrupting the client when necessary. To do this smoothly, it is vital that the counsellor gives the client a rationale for doing this and elicits their agreement to be interrupted.

Identify and understand the problem from the client's perspective

Single-session counsellors tend to be either solution-focused or problem- and solution-focused. If the counsellor is in the latter category, they must identify and understand the client's agreed problem from the client's perspective. Once the client 'feels' understood from their frame of reference, they will be more open to the counsellor's perspective than if they have not had that degree of empathy.

Assess the problem

Once the counsellor has communicated their understanding of the client's problem, they can assess it through the professional constructs they usually use and offer this to the client to see if it makes sense to them. If so, the counsellor and client can negotiate an agreed assessment of the problem that both can use going forward (Dryden, 2011).

Bridge to the future whenever possible

It is important to bring a future focus to the work in SSC. A client may want to discuss a past example of their nominated problem. However, as they will need to deal with the problem in the future, it may be better to have them identify and work with a predicted future example of the problem. Doing this encourages a smooth transition from the discussion of the problem and identification of the best solution to the implementation of this solution.

Use questions constructively

When I trained as a counsellor in the mid-1970s, we were strongly discouraged from asking our clients questions. To do so would mean we were operating from our frame of reference and not from that of our clients. However, most counsellors will find it impossible to practise SSC effectively without asking questions, particularly with a client who wants the counsellor to adopt a goal- and solution-focused stance. However, with a client who wants their counsellor to adopt a listening and/or exploratory role, the counsellor may well not use questions.[2]

Good practice when asking questions includes:

---

2. One of the most watched films about counselling features Carl Rogers counselling a client, 'Gloria', alongside Fritz Perls and Albert Ellis in the well-known *Three Approaches to Psychotherapy* series produced by Everett Shostrom in 1965. In the film, which may be found on YouTube, you can see how Rogers conducts a single session of counselling from a person-centred perspective and does so effectively without asking questions.

a) Ensure the client answers the questions they are asked.

If the counsellor is going to use questions in SSC, then it is vital to ensure, if possible, that the client answers the questions that the counsellor asks them. If the client does not answer an important question, then the counsellor needs to ask a different question to gain the information, if it is that important.

b) Give the client time to answer questions.

The SSC practitioner knows that they may only have one session with the client, so will be very conscious of how long they have for the work. However, to use that time effectively, it is important not to rush and to give the client enough time to think about the questions and formulate their answers.

Clarity

Clarity is a key factor in SSC and should characterise all the counsellor's communications with their client:

a) Whenever practicable, give an explanation for interventions.
One specific way in which the counsellor can demonstrate clarity is by explaining the major interventions they make with their client. This needs to be done, but it also needs to be done sparingly, not obsessively.

b) Make clear how the client can access further help.
Clarity is also key when the counsellor outlines for the client how they can access further help if needed. Ideally, this should be made clear at the beginning of the session and again at the end.

c) Check out the client's understanding of substantive points.
One way for the counsellor to check how clear they have been in their communications to the client is to check out the client's understanding of the salient points. Thus, the counsellor might say something like, 'I am not sure if I am making myself clear. Can you put into your own words the point you think I have been making?' The client's response may lead the counsellor to simplify the message.

Encourage the client to be as specific as possible but be mindful of opportunities for generalisation

The skilful SSC practitioner can range constructively along the continuum from the specific to the general when working with a client. The counsellor encourages the client to be specific when working with a salient example of their problem, in order to facilitate emotional processing, and encourages the client to generalise to other problems what they have learned from dealing with their nominated problem.

Identify and encourage the client to use salient strengths

SSC is founded on the central principle that the client has internal strengths that they can be helped to identify and use when addressing their nominated concern. It is crucial, therefore, that the counsellor asks the client to identify such strengths and finds ways of getting this information if the client denies having any such strengths. In these circumstances, the counsellor might ask the client such questions as:

- 'What would a close friend say your strengths are?'

- 'If you had applied for a job that you really wanted and were asked at interview what your strengths were as a person, what would you honestly say?'

- 'If you were in a really good frame of mind, what would you say that your strengths are?'

Once the client has identified some salient strengths, the counsellor helps them to identify how they can use the strengths to address their problem.

Identify and encourage the client to make use of salient aspects of their environment

The SSC practitioner also encourages the client to consider if there are factors in their environment that can also help them address their problem. For example, the client can be asked to consider which people in their life can support them while they are tackling their issue and how these people can best do this.

Identify previous attempts to solve their problem

It is quite likely that the client will have made several attempts to solve their problem in the past and it is important for the SSC practitioner to identify and understand these attempts:

a) Encourage the client to capitalise on successful attempts. If the client identifies previous problem-solving attempts that were successful, the counsellor helps both of them understand what was helpful about these attempts and encourages the client to use these elements in the future.

b) Discourage the client from using unsuccessful attempts. If the client mentions attempts to solve their problem that were ineffective, the counsellor helps them explore why they did not work and encourages them not to use them again in the future.

Undertake solution-focused work

The search for a solution is a key part of SSC, unless the client has indicated that they want to use the session to talk and be understood or to explore their concerns without searching for a solution. I see a solution as a response to the problem that enables the client to achieve their goal. The prime driver at this stage of the process is to encourage the client to identify a solution for themselves.

a) Offer the client expertise without assuming the role of expert. While the emphasis in solution-focused work is on encouraging the client to find a solution for themself, with the counsellor's active help, this does not mean that the counsellor cannot offer the client their perspective on what might constitute a solution to the client's problem. This is where insights from the counsellor's theoretical orientation may be useful. These should be offered to the client as *one* perspective on their problem and how it can be productively addressed, rather than *the* way to solve the problem.

b) Look for ways of making an emotional impact without pushing for it.

In searching for a solution, the counsellor should strive to engage the client's emotions so that the conversation can be meaningful for them. If the conversation is devoid of emotion, then the client will only engage intellectually with the counsellor; if the client is flooded with emotion, they will not be able to stand back and think about relevant matters.

c) Encourage the client to select a solution that they are most likely to implement.

The counsellor and client need, in my view, to be guided by pragmatism, rather than idealism, as they search for a solution that will help the client to address their problem effectively and achieve their goal. This means that, if an ideal solution exists, it should only be adopted if the client can implement it within the context of their life. If they are not able to do this, they should be encouraged to select a viable solution that they can implement and are willing to commit to.

d) Encourage the client to rehearse the solution in the session.

Once the client has selected a viable solution, the counsellor should encourage them to rehearse the solution in the session, if possible. The counsellor can suggest several ways in which the client can do this, including, imagery rehearsal, role-play, two-chair dialogue and behavioural rehearsal. Doing this helps the client to get a 'feel' of the solution to see if they can actually implement it, and to tweak it if necessary.

Encourage the client to take away just one thing

What the client takes away from the session is vital. There is some evidence from ongoing counselling that encouraging clients to take action based on what they have found valuable about the session increases the chances that they will do so (Jensen et al, 2019). In SSC, 'less is more', so the task of the counsellor is to help the client to nominate one such take-away.

My own experience in practising SSC is that, if I encourage the client to take away more from the session, they are less likely to act on it. From this, I have learned that it is better if my SSC clients leave the process with the 'one thing' that would make a difference to them (Keller & Papasan, 2012):

Have the client summarise the session

The client may be more likely to take away one meaningful thing from the session that they can implement later if the counsellor encourages them to summarise the session and what they have got from it, rather than summarising it for them. If the counsellor summarises the session, they are less likely to identify the client's take-away.

Help the client to develop an action plan

Once the client has identified a solution to their concern, practised it (if possible) and identified a relevant take-away,[3] they are ready to discuss how they are going to implement this learning. In ongoing counselling, this would take the form of a negotiated homework assignment – a specific task designed to help the person operationalise what they have learned in the session. However, in SSC, it is not known if the counsellor and client are going to meet again or, if they are, when that meeting might take place. Also, in one-at-a-time counselling, if the person does return, they may well see a different counsellor. For these reasons, it is more appropriate for the counsellor in SSC to help the client to develop a more general action plan, outlining the kinds of tasks that the client needs to carry out to reach their goal. These will be examples of the solution that the person developed with the counsellor earlier in the session.

---

3. It is better if the client's solution and takeaway are the same, since this conforms to the 'just one thing' principle that underpins SSC: the less the client takes away from the session, the more they are likely to remember and thus implement (Keller & Papasan, 2012). If the solution and take-away are different, the counsellor should help the client link them so they are combined into one point.

Here is an example. Jess was unhealthily angry about what she saw as her boss's unfair criticism of her work. Her *goal* was to stand up for herself with her boss without getting unhealthily angry. Her *solution* was two-fold:

- to first remind herself that her boss did not have to be fair to her, and then
- to assert herself and to request fairer treatment from him.

Her *action plan* was to approach her boss directly to seek feedback on her work, rather than avoid him (which she had been doing). She then planned to rehearse her new attitude and a self-assertion skill if she needed to do so.

Encourage the client to identify and problem-solve potential obstacles

Once the counsellor and client have agreed on an action plan, it would be nice to think that the client will definitely implement it. Some will, but others may encounter obstacles that lead them not to take action. As such, it is useful if the counsellor can ask the client to identify any potential obstacles to their implementing the action plan and then think about how they might respond to these obstacles, should they occur.

Identify and respond to the client's doubts, reservations and objections

As I mentioned earlier, the effectiveness of SSC is enhanced if the working alliance between the counsellor and client is strong (Simon et al, 2012). A critical aspect of the alliance is the views that the counsellor and client both hold about salient aspects of the process (Dryden, 2011). It is crucial that counsellor and client share a common perspective on these, so it is important for the counsellor to encourage the client to express any doubts, reservations and objections (DROs) to any aspect of the process. The client may communicate these DROs non-verbally, so the counsellor should be particularly alert to such expressions and respond accordingly. If the counsellor does this, at least they have an opportunity to respond to any misconceptions or misunderstandings that the client may have.

Tie up any loose ends

It is important that the session is brought to a proper conclusion, so the counsellor should seek to tie up any loose ends. This involves the counsellor:

- reminding the client how they may access future help, if needed
- inviting the client to ask any last-minute questions
- inviting the client to tell the counsellor anything they need to say before the close of the session.

Seek feedback from the client

Just before the client takes their leave, it is valuable for the counsellor to ask for feedback[4] about what they got from the session and what the counsellor could have done differently to help the person get more from the session.

It is also useful to get similar feedback after the client has had an opportunity to put into practice what they learned from the session and a reasonable amount of time has passed.

Bad practice in SSC

Simply reversing the above points will reveal what bad practice is in SSC. However, I would like to highlight some common counselling activities that, while helpful in other contexts, would be considered bad practice in SSC and are thus to be avoided.

---

4. The point at which you ask for feedback affects the feedback you get. In the so-called Pepsi Challenge, people preferred Pepsi to Coca-Cola when they were asked after takaing just a sip, largely because it is sweeter. When they were asked after having drunk more, the results tended to favour the less sweet beverage (Gladwell, 2005).

Avoid carrying out practices that yield information that is unnecessary for SSC

There are several common counselling practices that, while helpful in longer-term counselling, are not useful in SSC, given that they are time-consuming and do not yield very useful information. As noted in Chapter 7, these are:

- doing a full assessment of the client, including taking a case history and carrying out a case formulation
- taking a case history
- carrying out a case formulation.

Instead, the SSC practitioner should assess the client's nominated problem, how they have tried to address that problem and the internal strengths and external resources that they have at their disposal to deal with the issue.[5]

Avoid lack of structure, focus and direction

Earlier in this chapter, I argued that it is good practice for the counsellor to ask the client to indicate how they think the counsellor can best help them. Unless they say that the counsellor can help best by letting them talk in an unstructured way, the counsellor should give structure, direction and focus to the session. Thus, the counsellor should not let the client talk for long in an unfocused, general way. Also, the counsellor should not spend too much time in non-directive, listening mode, unless the client specifically asks them to do so. Further, a sense of direction is vital: if the counsellor does not encourage the client to identify a goal, neither the counsellor nor the client has anything to aim for. Finally, failure to bring the session to a satisfactory conclusion does not encourage the client to go away with a firm sense of purpose.

---

5. This applies to the SSC practitioner who is both problem- and solution-focused. The solution-focused single-session counsellor will forego problem assessment.

Avoid rushing

Practitioners who are pressured by the thought that they *only* have a finite amount of time in SSC are likely to rush the process and convey this sense of being pressured to the client. Consequently, the client may not think matters through with due consideration and will not derive as much benefit from the session as they would if a more relaxed SSC practitioner was helping them. For example, a counsellor who feels under such pressure is likely to ask their client multiple questions if the client does not answer their original question straight away. Asking a client multiple questions is frequently a sign of impatience and this quality will interfere significantly with the good practice of SSC.

In the next chapter, I will consider how SSC can be disseminated so that targeted client groups can learn about it and understand what it has to offer.

References

Bordin ES (1979). The generalizability of the psychoanalytic concept of the working alliance. *Psychotherapy: theory, research and practice 16*: 252–260.

Dryden W (2011). *Counselling in a Nutshell* (2nd ed). London: Sage.

Gladwell W (2005). *Blink: the power of thinking without thinking.* New York, NY: Little Brown & Company.

Jensen A, Fee C, Miles AL, Beckner DO, Persons JB (2019). Congruence of patient takeaways and homework assignment content predicts homework compliance in psychotherapy. *Behavior Therapy 51*(3): 424-433.

Keller G, Papasan J (2012). *The One Thing: the surprisingly simple truth behind extraordinary results.* Austin, TX: Bard Press.

Simon GE, Imel ZE, Ludman EJ, Steinfeld BJ (2012). Is dropout after a first psychotherapy visit always a bad outcome? *Psychiatric Services 63*(7): 705–707.

Chapter 9
Disseminating information about single-session counselling

Overview

Perhaps the most important issue that a counselling agency has to grapple with after they have decided to include SSC in their service delivery options is how to publicise it. How best do they communicate to their target population that SSC is now an option, what it is, who can benefit from it and how to access it.

In Chapter 7, I argued that, for SSC to thrive, it needs to have sufficient organisational and administrative support. One way to create this support is to invite stakeholders[1] to help the service develop dissemination material. Doing this helps all stakeholders to feel involved with the SSC service. So, in this chapter, I will consider *what* should be disseminated about SSC and *how* it should be disseminated.

---

1. A stakeholder in this context is anybody who has an interest in SSC as a way of delivering counselling. This would include the counsellors delivering the SSC service and relevant managers, supervisors of the counsellors, administrators of the service, representatives of service users and others who might have an involvement. Different agencies will have different views about which groups to involve and when. In my view, all relevant stakeholders need to be consulted about dissemination before the final information is made public, to ensure everyone feels included and consulted.

What information should be disseminated?[2]

To explore the material that should be disseminated about SSC, I will discuss the kind of information potential clients will want to know:

- how SSC should be described
- how people can access SSC
- the reasons a person should choose SSC
- the issues with which SSC can be helpful
- what SSC involves
- who provides SSC.

How should SSC be described?

It is unlikely that many potential clients will know what single-session counselling is, so the agency needs to make this clear in their dissemination material. My practice would be to make clear that it is a form of counselling and that it works best when the counsellor and client work with purpose, with the aim of helping the client in a single session while knowing that more help is available if needed.

This is how Relationships Australia Victoria (RAV) describes SSC on its website[3] and downloadable flyer:[4]

What is a single session consultation? A single-session consultation is an evidence-informed, client-focused

---

2. In outlining what information should be disseminated about SSC, I will draw on how one organisation, Relationships Australia Victoria (RAV), describes what it calls 'single session consultations'. RAV describes itself as a 'community-based, not-for-profit organisation, with no religious affiliations… Our objective is to relieve the suffering, distress and helplessness of vulnerable and disadvantaged people so as to enhance their physical, social and emotional wellbeing'.

3. See www.relationshipsvictoria.com.au/services/counselling/SSC/ (accessed 4 August 2019).

4. See www.relationshipsvictoria.com.au/assets/PDFs/Flyers/Single-Session-Consultations-flyer.pdf (accessed 4 August 2019).

counselling session. The focus of the session is on your greatest worry, challenge or difficulty, and what you want to achieve from your meeting. Our aim is for you to leave the session with some ideas or strategies to try out.

Single session consultations are suitable for individuals, couples or families. A single session consultation involves a longer than usual counselling session and a follow-up phone call to discuss the next steps.

Notice that RAV's description highlights the word 'consultation', rather than counselling, but that later it is referred to as a counselling session. It mentions SSC's evidence base, that it is focused on what the client deems to be their greatest difficulty, and that it is goal oriented. Then it mentions the counsellor's aim – for the client to leave with something to put into practice. Finally, it mentions the length of the session and that there will be a follow-up.

How can SSC be accessed?

It is vital for the dissemination material to make clear how potential clients can access SSC. In many university counselling services in the UK, where SSC is particularly popular, clients have to fill in an online form to access SSC. This form is available on the counselling service's website, with clear instructions about how to fill it in.

To use RAV as an example again, it offers clinical services at 12 locations, but only offers single-session consultations at two of them. This is made clear on its website and flyer. The email addresses and telephone numbers of the two locations appear on both the website and flyer. It is also made clear that attending a single session does not mean that the person cannot access RAV's other services.

Why a person should choose SSC

If a counselling agency offers several forms of counselling, it is useful to communicate the reasons why a person might wish to choose SSC over the other options. In my view, these reasons are:

- The person wants a rapid counselling response to their need. SSC may be delivered by walk-in or by appointment, but in both cases the response needs to be prompt
- The person wants to be helped in one session, with the knowledge that more sessions may be available.
- The person is able to focus on one issue at a time and wants to work with the issue they have chosen.

Here is what RAV says about this issue on its website.

Why should I choose a single session consultation?
People choose a single session consultation for different reasons. The sessions can help to make sure you're getting the most of your first, and sometimes only, session. Experience tells us about half the time people will come back for further counselling, while the rest are happy with one session. Both outcomes are okay. You are always welcome to return to RAV if you need further assistance.

In a single session consultation, our practitioners aim to make the most of your time by focusing on your greatest concern. Single session consultations are appealing because they are collaborative and responsive; they focus on your key concerns and goals, and you and your practitioner work together on strategies for change.

The RAV flyer is a little different, as can be seen below, presumably because there is less space:

Why should I choose an SSC? SSCs can help to make sure you're getting the most of your first, and sometimes only, session. SSCs are collaborative and responsive; they focus on your key concerns and goals, and you and your counsellor work together on strategies for change.

The issues with which SSC can be helpful

People who are considering SSC may be thinking about whether or not their concerns are suitable for this approach, so it is useful for an agency to outline the issues that people have tended to seek help for from SSC in the past. The downside to this is that, if a person's issue is not on the list, then they may not seek help from SSC when it might have been appropriate for them to have done so.

Here is what RAV says about this issue on their website and flyer:

For what issues can single session consultations be helpful? Single session consultations can be used for a wide range of issues. We work to help individuals, couples and families to improve their relationships and find ways to manage issues such as separation and divorce, grief and loss, mental health issues, life changes, family violence, managing emotions, parenting issues and managing stress.

The RAV SSC flyer ends at this point, but the website includes the following:

In fact, people attend single session consultations for the same reasons as ongoing counselling and other services. In a single session consultation, however, we can offer a contained and immediate response to your most pressing concern. While single session consultations focus on your greatest concern, they can still be suitable for those with multiple and/or complex issues. You may have a lot going on, but still find a single session to be helpful to you and your circumstances.

As can be seen from this, the RAV website covers the issue that I discussed above by reassuring people that any issue can be brought to SSC, even if it is complex and is not on the list of examples. Also, the website mentions that even people with multiple issues can benefit from SSC, where the focus will be on the person's most pressing concern.

What does SSC involve?

People need to know what SSC involves. There is the session itself: how long the session will last and who will be present. Also, if people are expected to complete any pre-session forms or go through other pre-session procedures, this needs to be made clear at this point. Information about follow-up should be included, as well as information about the possibilities for accessing future help, if needed.

Here is what RAV says about this issue on its website:

What does a single session consultation involve? Before you attend a session, you'll be sent a questionnaire to fill in, to help your practitioner find out more about your main concerns and goals for the session. You'll need to complete and return this questionnaire when you attend your session.

After your session, your counsellor will arrange a follow-up phone call to see how you're going and discuss options for further support. If you feel that the single session was sufficient and has met your needs, your practitioner will close your file, with the understanding you are welcome to re-contact RAV at any time in the future.

Note that there is nothing about what happens during the session itself.

The RAV flyer is, again, shorter on this point:

What happens during an SSC? Before you attend a session, you'll be sent a questionnaire to fill in, to help your counsellor find out more about your main concerns and goals for the session. After your session, your counsellor will arrange a follow-up phone call to see how you're going and discuss options for further support.

I think the heading here is a little confusing as the information given covers what happens before and after the consultation but not what happens during the consultation. It might have been better to use the same heading here as on the website: 'What does a single session consultation involve?'

Who provides SSC?

It is important for potential clients to know something about who will be offering SSC and, if relevant, what approach they bring to the work.

Here is what RAV says on its website and flyer about who provides SSCs:

> You will talk to one of our qualified counsellors who have extensive experience helping clients with a range of issues. Both male and female practitioners are available.

How should SSC be disseminated?

In the above section, I have focused on the 'what' of SSC information dissemination. In this section, I will focus on the 'how'.

Websites and flyers

In discussing the information about SSC disseminated by RAV, I drew from their website and a flyer explaining SSC. As we saw, on some issues, the flyer gave less information than the website because of space restrictions. My view is that, since websites can be accessed quite easily these days, the need for flyers may lessen, although counselling agencies should give due consideration to their target clientele on this point. For example, it is no good just using a website for dissemination purposes, if the target clientele cannot access the internet for information. For this client group, flyers or leaflets may be more appropriate.

2. Visual dissemination

If a picture is worth a thousand words, a moving picture is worth a lot more, so agencies should give due consideration to developing videos that explain SSC. This might involve counsellors first explaining who they are and then discussing issues such as:

- what SSC is
- what it involves
- why people should choose it
- the issues it can help with.

The video might include interviews with clients who have had SSC talking about how people can access it and their experiences of it. These videos can be posted on the agency's website and YouTube and uploaded on to other social media platforms.

Whiteboard animation[5] is another way of presenting information visually in a very simple format. These are animated sequences of images, with a script, that could be made both to promote an SSC service and to provide information about SSC more generally.[6]

Having discussed SSC dissemination, in the next chapter I will discuss the process of SSC.

5. See https://en.wikipedia.org/wiki/Whiteboard_animation (accessed 4 August 2019).

6. An example of a whiteboard animation to disseminate the general concept of SSC can be found at www.youtube.com/watch?v=wIcuOVOABRw (accessed 6 August 2019).

Chapter 10
The process of single-session counselling

Overview

In this chapter, I will consider the process of SSC from beginning to end. In doing so, I will draw heavily on the views of Michael Hoyt (2000, 2018). This chapter offers an overview of the material to be covered in Chapters 11 to 14.

It is sometimes thought that a single session of counselling involves concertinaing several sessions into one (see Chapter 15). Nothing could be further from the truth. The single session has a process of its own and comprises six phases:

1. Before the client and counsellor agree to work together in SSC

2. The pre-session preparation phase, once the client and counsellor have decided to work together in SSC

3. The early phase of the session

4. The middle phase of the session

5. The late phase of the session

6. The follow-through phase.

The competent SSC practitioner keeps these phases in mind while working with the client, before during and after the session.

Phase 1: Before the client and counsellor agree to work together in SSC

What happens before the client and counsellor opt for SSC can be seen as phase 1 of the SSC process. It may be helpful to think of four help-seeking roles that the person can occupy (Garvin & Seabury, 1997; Dryden, 2019):

- the explorer
- the enquirer
- the applicant
- the client.

The explorer role

In the 'explorer' role, the person is interested in counselling and is exploring the varied different modes of counselling on offer, including SSC. In their exploration, they may have identified an agency that offers SSC and may have read what is published on that agency's website and in its written literature. They may have identified counsellors who practise SSC, as well as those who offer brief or longer-term counselling. However, they have not yet approached any agency or counsellor.

The enquirer role

The 'enquirer' will have concluded that SSC might help them and will have begun to find out about particular agencies or counsellors who offer it. The enquiries may range from the technical, seeking more detailed information about how the agency or counsellor operates, to the practical, such as fees, if any, and how help can be accessed. Sometimes this information will be available on an agency's website.

The applicant role

The 'applicant' has decided that SSC will help them, has identified the agency or counsellor they think is best suited to them and has made an appointment for SSC or asked the counsellor if they will take them on for SSC.

The client role

An applicant for SSC becomes a client when they have understood the nature of SSC and have given their informed consent to proceed (Garvin & Seabury, 1997). This consent indicates that both counsellor and client understand their respective tasks and agree to carry these out. Crucially, it involves the client understanding what help, if any, is available after the session.

Phase 2: The pre-session preparation phase

As I have already mentioned, SSC can be accessed by walk-in or by appointment. If the person seeks SSC at a walk-in centre, there will usually be a short waiting period between walking in and seeing a counsellor. During this gap, the person can be asked to complete a pre-session form to enable them and their counsellor to get the most from the session. I will discuss this more fully in the next chapter.

If the person seeks SSC by appointment, there will of course be a longer time between the request for SSC and the appointment date, but hopefully not too long. During that period, the person can be asked to complete a pre-session form or take part in a telephone conversation with the counsellor to help both prepare themselves for the work and ensure the client gains maximum benefit from the session. Such pre-session contact can also be used to help introduce the client to SSC and plant the seeds for change.

Phase 3: The early phase of the session

We have now reached the stage where the client and counsellor first meet in person. The counsellor begins the session by clarifying with the client the purpose of their meeting and making clear at the outset how they can access further help if needed.

At the outset, the counsellor explores whether the client has experienced any change in the issue for which they are seeking help and, if so, they can build on this change. In this early phase of the session, the counsellor sets out to form a productive working alliance with the client and demonstrates their keenness to help the client as quickly as possible. The counsellor encourages the client to identify a goal for the session and, if they are problem- and solution-focused, they strive to understand the client's problem and link it with their nominated goal.

Phase 4: The middle phase of the session

In the middle phase of the session, the counsellor works with the client to effect change in the factor that is responsible for the continuation of the client's problem. It is crucial here that counsellor and client agree what this factor is (Dryden, 2011). How it is changed depends on several issues: first, the client's view of how it can be best changed and to what; second, what the client has tried before to achieve this change, what has worked and what has not, and third, what concepts specific to their therapeutic orientation the counsellor brings to the conversation.

On this point, it is best if the counsellor has asked the client if they are interested in the counsellor's perspective on the issue before they introduce it. The agreed solution emerges from a discussion of these points. Then, the client and counsellor discuss the practicality of the solution as well as its likely effectiveness in effecting the desired change.[1]

Once a solution has been agreed, the counsellor suggests that the client rehearses the solution in the session, if possible, to get some experience in implementing it. If, based on this experience, the client concludes that the solution is not right for them, the counsellor and client can choose another solution and rehearse it. If the client concludes that the first solution is right for them, they still can make some changes to the solution, if necessary.

---

1. It is important to note here that the most effective solution may not be the most practicable. Thus, the counsellor should preferably help the person to select a solution that they will implement even if it is less therapeutically powerful than another solution that the client will not implement.

Phase 5: The late phase of the session

In the late phase of SSC, the counsellor and client discuss how the client can implement the solution that they have selected and rehearsed earlier in the session. The discussion will centre on action planning, where the client decides on a *broad* strategy of implementation. While specific examples of such action planning may be identified, mainly to help the client kick start the process, the emphasis needs to be on one primary, broad implementation principle. The counsellor can then ask the client to identify and problem-solve any obstacles to the implementation of their action plan.

The counsellor can also ask the client to summarise what they learned from the session that they will take away with them. The counsellor should find ways to link together the client's solution, how they plan to implement it and their take-away, if these are different.

Once this has been done, the client can begin to wrap things up. During this part of the process, the counsellor should encourage the client to ask any last-minute questions and/or make any final points before plans for follow-up are made. They should repeat that the client may access further help if needed and clarify how.

At the end of this late phase, the client should leave the session on a positive note, optimistic that they can operationalise meaningful learning from the session.

Phase 6: The follow-through phase

The follow-through phase involves the counsellor (or the counsellor's representative) following up the client at an agreed date after the session. The purpose of this follow-up is two-fold: first, to discover the longer-term outcome of the session for the client (outcome evaluation), and second, to find out from the client what they thought about the service they received (service evaluation). This is a good time for the client to indicate if they need further help, if they haven't already asked for it or said they don't need it.

References

Dryden W (2019). *Single-Session Coaching and One-At-A-Time Coaching: distinctive features.* Abingdon: Routledge.

Dryden W (2011). *Counselling in a Nutshell* (2nd ed). London: Sage.

Garvin CD, Seabury BA (1997). *Interpersonal Practice in Social Work: promoting competence and social justice* (2nd ed). Boston, MA: Allyn & Bacon.

Hoyt MF (2018). Single-session therapy: stories, structures, themes, cautions, and prospects. In: Hoyt MF, Bobele M, Slive A, Young J, Talmon J, Talmon M (eds). *Single-Session Therapy by Walk-In or Appointment: administrative, clinical, and supervisory aspects of one-at-a-time services.* New York, NY: Routledge (pp155–174).

Hoyt MF (2000). *Some Stories are Better than Others: doing what works in brief therapy and managed care.* Philadelphia, PA: Brunner/Mazel.

Chapter 11
Helping clients prepare for and get the most from single-session counselling

Overview

In this chapter, I will explore ways in which clients be helped to prepare for and get the most from SSC. I will describe the major elements of such preparation. I will discuss its four main foci:

- its problem focus

- its future, goal-directed focus

- its focus on important *internal* factors

- its focus on important *external* variables.

I will also discuss briefly how to use the pre-session contact to plant the seed of change.

Introduction

The growing interest in SSC can be traced to the publication of Moshe Talmon's (1990) book *Single-Session Therapy: maximising the effect of the first (and often only) therapeutic encounter.* This book also addresses what exactly SSC is (see also Chapter 1 in this book). Does SSC involve one contact and one contact only, which in Chapter 1 I refer to as the 'Ronseal' definition of SSC (Dryden, 2019)? Does SSC encompass a pre-session contact? Can SSC refer to counselling that takes place one session at a time and does not involve booking 'blocks' of counselling sessions?

Clearly, if SSC is one contact only (as in walk-in counselling), this precludes the client from preparing themself for the session other than by filling in a pre-session form just before they receive SSC. Even if they do this, they will have little time to digest the questions that they have been asked to answer.

Thus, it is only in SSC by appointment that the client can prepare thoroughly for the face-to-face session.[1] This preparation can take place by telephone or by completing a pre-session form that is returned to the counsellor with enough time for them to digest the information and prepare themself for the session. The advantage of the pre-session telephone conversation is that it is interactive, so the counsellor can react to the person's previous answers and draw links between different elements of what the client has said. The advantage of the pre-session form is that the client can take their time to complete it and can stop and restart it at their leisure. Perhaps the best of both worlds would be for the client to complete the pre-session form first and then have a pre-session telephone conversation with the counsellor that is focused on their responses. This would enable the counsellor to help the client reflect on more focused information before the face-to-face session.

What follows is a discussion of the questions asked during the pre-session phase of SSC.

Problem focus

Counsellors in SSC tend to be solution-focused in that they are keen to help their clients deal quickly with their problems.

1. In this book, I am mainly discussing SSC that takes place face-to-face between counsellor and client. However, it is important to note that modern-day counselling can also take place online by Skype or through text messaging.

Counsellors may also be problem-focused, and if so, they need to help the client focus on the main problem for which they are seeking help. Given this, the client can be asked a focusing question such as:

- 'What is the one problem or concern that seems most important to focus on now?'

Relevant information about the problem

It is useful for the counsellor to know a little about the problem. What is relevant will largely be determined by the client, and so it is useful to start by asking the client a question such as:

- 'What do you think I need to know about the problem to be able to help you with it?'

One useful piece of information is the reason for seeking help now:

- 'What made you decide that now was the right time to seek help?'

If the client does not indicate the impact of the problem on their life, the counsellor can ask:

- 'How does the problem affect you and/or other people in your life?'

Previous attempts to address the problem

It is important for both counsellor and client to understand what the client has done previously to address the problem so that the client can be helped to capitalise on helpful strategies and let go of unhelpful ones. Thus, the following questions are useful:

- 'What have you tried that has helped you with this problem?'
- 'What have you tried that has not helped with the problem or made it worse?'

The counsellor's helping stance

While the counsellor will have their own ideas about how they can be helpful to the client, what is equally vital, or perhaps even more so, is:

- 'How do you think I can best help you deal with the problem?'

Future, goal-directed focus

SSC has a future, goal-directed focus, but one that is more immediate than in longer-term counselling. This immediate focus is reflected in the following questions:

- 'What would you like to get out of the session?'

- 'How will you know when you have achieved the changes you desire?'

Focus on important internal factors

SSC is a mode of counselling delivery that relies greatly on the client drawing on a number of pre-existing inner factors or qualities. The SSC's skill lies in helping the client to identify and use these factors.

It is useful to begin the focus on client factors by helping the client to see themself as an efficacious solver of personal problems. To this end, the counsellor can ask:

- 'Remember a problem that happened any time in your life that you resolved in such a way that left you feeling proud of yourself. What did you do that you felt proud of?

Identifying and using inner strengths

Next, the counsellor needs to help the client to identify their inner strengths by asking:

- 'What strengths as a person do you have that will help you deal with the problem effectively?'

If the client struggles to answer this direct question, alternatives might be:

- 'What would people who know you really well say in answer to the same question?'

- 'If you went to an interview for a job you really wanted and you were to name your genuine strengths as a person, what would you say?'

Once the client has identified their strengths, they can be asked how they can use them in addressing their problem:

- 'How do you think you can use these strengths to solve your problem?'

Other internal factors

There are a number of other internal factors that may be useful to find out about. If the counsellor is carrying out a pre-session telephone conversation, they may be selective about what to ask, depending on what was discussed earlier. On the pre-session form, it is not known what might be relevant, so they may enquire about all such factors.

- **Core values.** 'What core values do you have that you and I might refer to in addressing your problem?'

- **Role models.** 'Who do you consider to be a role model who might directly or indirectly be helpful to you as you address your problem?'

- **Preferred way of learning.** 'I would like to know your preferred way of learning so that I can tailor the session to best help you. How do you best like to earn?'

Focus on important external factors

In addition to the internal factors, it is useful for the client to be asked about aspects of their environmental, external factors that they can use to good effect in SSC. The counsellor might ask:

- 'Which people in your life right now could help and/or support you as you address the problem?'
- 'Are there any organisations that can help you address your problem?'

Other issues

With no contextual information, it is difficult for the counsellor to know what other issues they might find useful to know about, so they might ask the client:

- 'For me to be most helpful, is there anything you feel is important for me to know about your culture, ethnicity, religion, language, sexual orientation, gender identity/expression, mental or physical health, or other factor?'

Planting the seed of change

Since the counsellor is having some pre-session contact with the client, it may be useful for them to plant a seed of change with them. To this end, some counsellors use de Shazer's (1985) concept of the 'skeleton key' (Talmon, 1990), in the following instruction:

- 'Between now and our face-to-face session, I would like you to notice the things that happen to you that you would like to keep happening in the future, relevant to the problem. In this way, you will help us to find out more about your goal.'

Table 11.1 provides the questions discussed above in a form that clients can complete and counsellors can use while conducting the pre-session telephone conversation. In this situation, the counsellor can make notes in the appropriate spaces. These questions are only suggestions; the form/telephone call protocol can be modified to suit the individual client.

Table 11.1: Pre-session questionnaire

1. What is the one problem or concern that seems most important to focus on now?

2. What do you think I need to know about the problem to be able to help you with it?

3. What made you decide that now was the right time to seek help?

4. How does the problem affect a) you? b) other people in your life?

5. What have you tried that has helped you with this problem?

6. What have you tried that has not helped with the problem or made it worse? How do you think I can best help you deal with the problem?

7. What would you like to get out of the session?

8. How will you know when you have achieved the changes you desire?

9. Remember a problem that happened at any time in your life that you resolved in such a way that left you feeling proud of yourself. What did you do that you felt proud of?

10. What strengths as a person do you have that will help you deal with the problem effectively?

11. If the client struggles to answer this direct question, alternatives are:
    - What would people who know you really well say in answer to the same question?
    - If you went to an interview for a job you really wanted and you were to name your genuine strengths as a person, what would you say?

12. How do you think you can use such strengths to solve your problem?

13. What core values do you have that you and I might refer to in our work together in addressing your problem?

14. Who do you consider to be a role model who might directly or indirectly be helpful to you as you address your problem?

15. I would like to know your preferred way of learning so that I can tailor the session to help you best. How do you best like to learn?

16. Who in your life right now could support you as you address the problem?

17. For me to be most helpful, is there anything you feel is important for me to know about your culture, ethnicity, religion, language, sexual orientation, gender identity/ expression, mental or physical health or any other factor?

18. Between now and our face-to-face session, I would like you to notice the things that happen to you that you would like to keep happening in the future that are relevant to the problem. In this way, you will help us to find out more about your goal.

When the pre-session contact may be enough

Sometimes it happens that, after completing the pre-session contact form or having the pre-session telephone call, the person decides that they do not need the session. There may be several reasons for this. First, the person may realise, in the course of completing the form or after having had the telephone conversation with the counsellor, that they need a different service, not SSC. However, my experience is that, more often, going through the form or interview leads the person to realise that they can address the issue on their own. For example, several people have told me after our pre-session telephone conversation that my questions led them to recognise that they do have the wherewithal to address the problem and that they can ask one of their friends, for example, to help them. Apparently, any contact with a helper can be therapeutic in this respect.

In the next chapter, I will discuss what is covered in a single session of counselling.

References

de Shazer S (1985). *Keys to Solution in Brief Therapy.* New York, NY: WW Norton & Co.

Dryden W (2019). *Single-Session Therapy: 100 key points and techniques.* Abingdon: Routledge.

Talmon M (1990). *Single-Session Therapy: maximising the effect of the first (and often only) therapeutic encounter.* San Francisco, CA: Jossey-Bass.

Chapter 12
What is covered in single-session counselling?

Overview

In this chapter, I will discuss what tends to be covered in the face-to-face session of SSC. I will assume that the client and counsellor have not had any pre-session contact, as quite often this is the case. However, I will suggest, at relevant points, what the counsellor can do when the two have had pre-session contact. I will discuss issues to do with beginning the session, dealing with the nominated problem, focusing and effecting change and bringing the session to a satisfactory conclusion.

Before I do so, I want to make a two related points. First, what follows is not a manual to which the counsellor should strictly adhere. Rather, it is a map to guide the counsellor at various points in the session. Second, in the same way as a maintenance worker does not use all the tools in their toolbox while undertaking a specific job, the counsellor will not use all of the guidelines outlined in this chapter. They are presented here so the counsellor knows they can draw on a range of strategies and techniques during a session, as needed.

Beginning the session

There are several issues that the counsellor needs to clarify with the client at the start of the session.

Explain the service that the client is being offered

When the counsellor and client first meet, it is important that the counsellor makes clear what the client is being offered and ensures that they want it. This should be done even if the counsellor and client have had pre-session contact. The counsellor needs to make clear whether it is possible for the client to access future help and how this can be done. However, the emphasis should be on helping the client in the one session that they know they are going to have together.

Explain confidentiality

As in any form of counselling, the counsellor needs to explain the principle of confidentiality and to make clear the exceptions to absolute confidentiality.

Obtain informed consent

Once the client has understood and agreed to SSC and what the counsellor has told them about confidentiality, they can be regarded as having given their informed consent to proceed. They can give their consent verbally or in writing.

Refer to and capitalise on the pre-session contact

If the counsellor has had pre-session contact with the client, it is useful for the counsellor to refer to it at the beginning of the session and capitalise on it, if possible. This is particularly the case if the two have had an interactive pre-session telephone conversation, or if the client has completed the written pre-session contact form and sent it to the counsellor so that they have had a chance to digest it.

There are several ways in which the counsellor can refer to the pre-session contact. Some examples include:

1.   If the counsellor suggested the 'skeleton key' exercise (see

Chapter 11), then they might ask the client what changes they have noticed following the session. If they have noticed a change, then the counsellor can use this information to help the person set a goal and move towards it.

2.   In making a general connection between the pre-session contact and the session, the counsellor can ask the client if they have had any thoughts since the pre-session contact that might help them both in the session.

Establish the focus

To get the most from SSC, it is important for the counsellor and client to use the time they have together in a way that the client deems productive. They need to agree on this quite quickly.

How can I best help you?

Asking the client how they think the counsellor can best help them is a good first step to establish a focus for the session. Mostly, clients nominate a problem for which they would like help, but sometimes a client may say that they want the counsellor to listen to them while they talk, or they want the counsellor to help them to explore a particular area. In this case, the two of them agree to it, and this becomes the focus of the session.

What is the single most important concern that you have right now?

A common focus in SSC is a particular issue with which the person needs help. When the person has only one problem, the focus is simple, so long as the problem is within the client's control to resolve. If the person wants to change another person, that is more problematic. If this is the case, the counsellor should help the client distinguish between changing another person (which is not within their control) and making attempts to influence the other (which is more within their control, since they are making the attempts). If the latter focus is chosen, then the counsellor still needs to help the person see that their attempts to influence might fail and, if this happens, they need to accept (but not like) the grim reality that the other person may not change. This acceptance is a prelude to a discussion about the person's options in such an eventuality.

When the client mentions several problems, as previously highlighted, it is important for the counsellor to encourage them to focus on one of them. However, having helped the client to prioritise the primary problem, the counsellor still needs to be mindful of their other needs. This means, later in the session, helping the client to see the connection between their problems, if relevant.

Explore the most important type of help needed

I mentioned above that, before a focus has been agreed, the counsellor can ask the client how best they think the counsellor can help them. Once the focus of the session has been agreed, then the counsellor can ask the client a more specific question, such as, 'What help do you need to deal with the problem?'

Check the focus

Once the counsellor and client have agreed on a focus for the session, it is important for the counsellor to check with the client at various points in the session to determine whether or not the client is still talking about what they think is the most relevant issue for them. If not, the counsellor facilitates a shift to a new, more relevant focus.

Maintain the focus

Even if the nominated focus is the most relevant, the client may still wander from it. Before this happens, it is helpful if the counsellor says something like, 'Sometimes, even after we have agreed a focus, you may move away from it. If this happens, may I have your permission to interrupt and bring you back to the focus?' In my experience, the client will readily give permission, observing that they do tend to wander and would appreciate being brought back by the counsellor.

Assess risk

When I give workshops on SSC to university counselling services, one of the most frequent questions asked by participants concerns the management of risk in the single session. By risk, they mean when the client is at immediate risk of suicide or harming themself or others. My response is that the counsellors should do in SSC exactly what they would do in other forms of counselling. The one thing that may be different is that, given the emphasis in SSC on providing help at the point of need, the counsellor is likely to find out earlier in SSC if the client is at risk and so they (the client) would get the help they need quicker too.

Dealing with the nominated problem

As previously stated, SSC practitioners are either solution-focused or problem- and solution-focused. In this section, I will discuss how problem- and solution-focused counsellors help clients to deal with their nominated problem (ie. the one problem or issue that the client and counsellor have agreed to focus on during the session).

Understand the problem

When striving to understand the problem, the SSC practitioner may elicit the client's understanding of the problem or offer their conceptualisation,[1] or both. Since the single-session counsellor tends to be pluralistic in outlook,[2] they will tend to do both and work towards a negotiated viewpoint. As we have seen, this tends to strengthen the working alliance (see Chapter 8), which in turn is associated with a better outcome for the client (Dryden, 2011; Simon et al, 2012).

---

1. It is here that counsellors may bring insights from their preferred therapeutic orientation.

2. By which I mean that they are open to multiple perspectives on the same clinical phenomena and tend to privilege the client's perspective (Cooper & McLeod, 2011; Cooper & Dryden, 2016).

Identify problem-creating and problem-maintaining factors

One way of conceptualising why a person has a problem is that they have responded to a negative situation[3] with a set of factors that create and maintain the problem. This is shown in Figure 12.1.

Figure 12.1: From adversity to problem

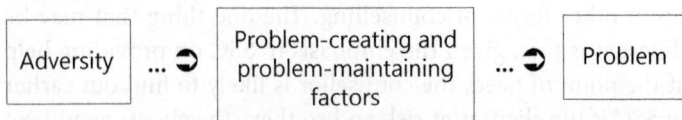

From this perspective, it is important for the counsellor and client to understand these problem-creating and problem-maintaining factors, since they may need to be addressed during the session.

Discover and use the client's previous attempts to deal with the problem

People usually try to resolve a problem themselves. Given this, the counsellor needs to discover from the client how they have previously attempted to deal with the problem. If this information has been obtained from the pre-session contact, it can be reviewed at this point. If not, the counsellor can ask:

• 'What have you tried in the past that has helped with the problem?'

It may be that what the client deemed to be helpful was only helpful to them in the short term. However, they may have used strategies that had some positive impact in the longer term. If so, they can be encouraged to use these as counsellor and client work towards finding a solution to the client's problem later in the session. They can also ask:

---

3. In this book, I refer to this negative situation as an adversity (Dryden, 2016).

- 'What have you tried in the past that has not helped with the problem?'

The client should be discouraged from using these strategies going forward, even though they may have become habitual.

Focusing on and effecting change

Focusing on and effecting change is a crucial part of the single session. It involves helping the client to:

- set a realistic goal for the session
- identify and use inner strengths and resiliency factors, as well as external resources
- review potential change factors
- identify potential solutions that will help the client to achieve their goal, using all the above factors, and select the one that is most practicable and likely to effect change
- have the client practise the solution in the session, if practicable
- develop an action plan
- identify and address any potential obstacles to implementing the plan.

Set a realistic goal for the session

All the client and counsellor know for certain is that they will be meeting for the one session they are currently having. Because of that, the counsellor asks the client what they would like to achieve by the end of the session, rather than by the end of counselling, which is more customary. In doing so, the counsellor advises the client to set a goal that is realistic and helps them to do this.

Identify and use inner strengths and resiliency factors

As there is not enough time for the counsellor to teach the client new skills, it is important that the two work with the client's strengths and resiliency factors in constructing a solution. With the problem in mind, the client should be asked to nominate which of their identified strengths and/or resiliency factors they might use in constructing a potential solution to the problem that may help them to achieve their goal. Once this has been done, the counsellor has a conversation with the client concerning *how* they use these inner factors to this end. It is important, therefore, for the client to nominate specific examples of such goal-directed behaviour.

What to do if the client struggles to identify strengths and resiliency factors

If the client struggles to identify strengths and resiliency factors, it is important that the counsellor gives them more information to enable them to do so. I normally say that a *strength* is something that the client is good at (eg. persistence, being creative), a positive character trait that they have[4] (eg. honesty or loyalty) or a healthy attitude (being hopeful or having a sense of personal control. I normally say that a *resiliency factor* is something that helps them withstand adversity (eg. religious or spiritual conviction or tolerating discomfort). I then give the client examples of how such strengths and resiliency factors may serve as important components in problem-solving.

This educative work generally helps the client to identify their own strengths and/or resiliency factors.

Identify and use external resources

The client's internal factors are not the only resource that the client can make use of in SSC. They can also use external resources to help themselves. One concept that I apply in this respect is that of 'team', as in, 'Who is on your team?'[5] Thus, the counsellor can ask the client, 'Which people on your team can help you as you address your problem and what help and/or support can they provide?'

---

4. Thus, we speak of strength of character.

5. The term 'team' in this context means anyone in the client's life to whom they can turn for help and/or support.

Examples of other external resources to which the client can turn are organisations, apps and self-help books. It is useful if the client can be helped to see what specific assistance they can get from a specific external resource.

Identify potential change factors

As the phrase indicates, 'change factors' are factors that the client can use in developing a solution to their problem. These include the inner strengths, resiliency factors and external resources discussed above. They also include constructive alternatives to the problem-maintaining factors discussed earlier in the chapter.

It is here that the counsellor may again bring to the session ideas that come from their favoured therapeutic orientation. In my workshops on SSC, I argue that SSC can be practised by counsellors from a range of different therapeutic orientations. That is why there is no manual on how to practise SSC, since it can be practised in different ways as long as the counsellor has the SSC mindset.

Identify the solution

As Figure 12.2 shows, a solution is a response to the same adversity that features in the person's problem but one that leads the person to achieve their goal. A good way of opening the discussion on this issue is by asking questions such as:

* 'What would be the smallest change needed to show you that things are heading in the right direction?'

* 'From what we have discussed so far what would best help you to solve your problem?'

Figure 12.2: From adversity to goal

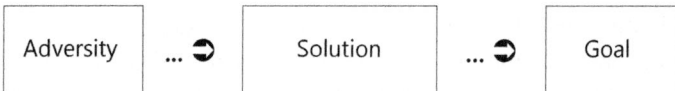

In searching for a solution, it is important for both counsellor and client to bear in mind both the potential effectiveness and the practicality of the solution. A client will not implement an effective solution that is not practicable, and there is no point in them implementing a practicable solution that will not be effective.

Encourage the practice of the solution in the session

Once a solution that is both potentially effective and practicable has been co-constructed by the counsellor and client, the counsellor should, ideally, encourage the client to practise the solution, if possible. The purpose of this is to enable the client to get some first-hand experience of what it is like to implement the solution. Two outcomes are possible. If the practice leads the person to conclude that the solution is not right for them, then the counsellor can help them to discover a different solution, which again needs to be practised, if there is time. If the practice leads the person to conclude that the solution is right for them, it gives them the opportunity to fine-tune the solution on the basis of that practice.

Develop an action plan

Once the client has practised the solution and has made some modifications as described above, the counsellor encourages them to develop a plan to put the solution into practice. This plan should be expressed in general terms so that it can guide the specific implementation of the solution in specific and relevant contexts. It is a good idea for the counsellor to help the client to put the solution into operation as soon after the session as possible, to 'kick start' the action plan.

Identify and address any potential obstacles

Once the client has been helped to develop their action plan, it is good practice for the counsellor to help the client to identify any obstacles that can potentially derail them from implementing the solution. Once they are identified, it is useful for the counsellor to help the client to specify how they would deal with the obstacles in advance.

Bringing the session to a satisfactory close

Once the client has done some advanced problem-solving concerning dealing with potential obstacles to change, the counsellor should begin to bring the session to a close. This involves the following tasks.

Ask the client to summarise what they will take away from the session

At the end of the session, the counsellor might be tempted to summarise what was discussed in the session. They should resist the temptation. It is better to ask the client to provide the summary, and particularly what they will be taking away from the process.[6] There are two main reasons why the counsellor should ask the client to provide the summary. The first is that, otherwise, the counsellor will not know what the client take-away is. The second is that it encourages the client to remain active in the process, even at the end.

Ideally, as discussed in Chapter 8, the client take-away should be synonymous with the solution; if not, the counsellor should help link the two for the client.

Encourage closure

It is important that the client leaves the session with hope and a sense of closure. With respect to the latter, the counsellor might ask the following questions:

- 'What question(s) might you wish you had asked me when you get home today? Please ask them now.'

- 'Is there anything you would like me to know that you have not told me before we finish? Please tell me now.'

In my experience, both can be dealt with quite quickly and links made with what was discussed in the session, if appropriate.

---

6. This is known as a client take-away (Jensen et al, 2019).

Revisit the issue of further help

Earlier in this chapter, I said that, at the start of the session, the counsellor should clarify with the client whether further help is available, and if so, how it can be accessed. This issue should be revisited at the end of the session.

Explain the reflect-digest-action-wait-decide process

In Chapter 1, I discussed the concept of 'one-at-a-time' counselling and explained that a central part of this is encouraging the client to reflect on and digest what they learned from the session, take action based on that learning and see what happens before deciding whether or not to make another appointment. The counsellor might invite the client to engage in this five-stage process or give it as one option at the end of the session. Thus, a counsellor might say something like:

- 'At this point, there are two ways to progress. First, you might want to make another appointment now. Second, you may want to reflect on what you have learned, digest this learning, put this learning into practice and see what happens before making a decision about making another appointment. Both approaches are equally valid. Which would suit you best?'

If the client expresses a wish to book a further session, then the counsellor should let them know how they can do this, and whether it can be with them or with another counsellor (if applicable), and refer them back to whoever makes the appointments.

Arrange follow-up

Before closing the session, the last matter to be dealt with is arranging a follow-up with the client, if applicable. I will discuss this issue in greater depth in Chapter 14. For now, I will say that, if it has been agreed that there will be a follow-up, the counsellor and client need to agree a date, who will initiate contact and how this will be done.

In the next chapter, I will present a verbatim transcript of SSC with commentary to show how one single-session counsellor works.

References

Cooper M, Dryden W (eds) (2016). *The Handbook of Pluralistic Counselling and Psychotherapy.* London: Sage.

Cooper M, McLeod J (2011). *Pluralistic Counselling and Psychotherapy.* London: Sage.

Dryden W (2016). *Attitudes in Rational Emotive Behaviour Therapy: components, characteristics and adversity-related consequences.* London: Rationality Publications.

Dryden W (2011). *Counselling in a Nutshell* (2nd ed). London: Sage.

Jensen A, Fee C, Miles AL, Beckner DO, Persons JB (2019). Congruence of patient takeaways and homework assignment content predicts homework compliance in psychotherapy. *Behavior Therapy 51*(3): 424-433.

Simon GE, Imel ZE, Ludman EJ, Steinfeld BJ (2012). Is dropout after a first psychotherapy visit always a bad outcome? *Psychiatric Services 63*(7): 705–707.

Chapter 13
What does a single session of counselling look like?

Overview

In the previous chapter, I discussed what can be covered in SSC and stressed that not all the points raised will necessarily be present in every session of SSC. In this chapter, I will present the transcript of a single session that I carried out in the context of giving a workshop on SSC.

Introduction

It is important that you get a sense of how SSC can be practised. However, it is also important that you appreciate that SSC can be practised in different ways, so I am not holding up this session as a model to be followed. All I am doing is showing how I, as a practitioner, worked with one client. I will provide comments at salient points of the session and conclude the chapter by outlining eight elements of my SSC practice that the session demonstrates.

How I practise single-session counselling

The following session took place during a one-day workshop that I was giving on SSC and was the second of two demonstration sessions I did that day. When I ask for a volunteer in this setting, I stress that the person needs to have a genuine current emotional problem with which they would like help and which they don't mind discussing in front of an audience of their peers. The person has given me their written permission to use the transcript included here and asked that I use the name 'Shell Annette' when referring to her. What follows is the transcript of this session, with my commentary.

The session

Windy: OK, Shell Annette, what problem can I help you with today?

Shell Annette: It's anxiety. My anxiety is absolutely through the roof.

Windy: Is it?

Shell Annette: Yeah... I feel that I've just got no time for me. And I notice when I talk, the urgency all the time in my voice: 'I need to do this,' 'I've got to do this.' I just feel like I'm on a timer all the time to do everything.

I am immediately aware that Shell Annette has voiced a number of rigid attitudes that might account for her anxiety. Such attitudes tend to underpin a range of emotional problems, and it is a concept that I, as a practitioner of rational emotive behaviour therapy (REBT), tend to bring to SSC (Dryden, 2016).

Windy: OK. And, so, when you volunteered to come up here today, what was that for?

Shell Annette: Me. That was for me.

Windy: Right. So, you've made a start to do something for you.

Right from the start, I am looking for ways to encourage change. Shell Annette says that she has no time for herself, and yet she has done something for herself by volunteering for help. I make this point explicitly.

Shell Annette: Yeah.

Windy: How did you manage to decide to do that, because you could have not volunteered?

Shell Annette: I couldn't stop my hand going up. I thought, 'Don't put it up!' because I'm not very good at talking in groups. I don't like being up front, but I just thought, 'Do you know, just push yourself through that.'

Windy: Push yourself through the…?

Shell Annette: Through the fear.

Windy: Right.

Shell Annette: Because my heart's absolutely palpitating right now.

Windy: Is it?

Shell Annette: Yeah. I'm shaking.

Windy: Right. So, you've made the decision to do something for yourself.

Shell Annette: Yes.

Windy: Even though it felt like your hand had a life of its own.

Shell Annette: Yes.

Windy: And, even though you are feeling quite anxious right now, you decided to come up and do it anyway.

I am emphasising the point here that it is possible to choose to do something to help oneself despite being anxious.

Shell Annette: Yes.

Windy: OK, alright. So, what do you take from that?

Shell Annette: … That I'm probably braver than I actually think I am.

Windy: And by braver, you mean what?

Shell Annette: [Pause] I think, for a lot of years, I thought I was stupid and thick and I put myself down. And I've learnt, over the past couple of years, or few years while I've been doing the counselling training, that actually I'm not quite that stupid; I can do things.

Windy: You can do things and you're brave. OK. So, tell me a little bit about, if you, again, were to leave here thinking that, 'I'm pleased that I actually volunteered to talk about that,' what would you have realistically achieved as a result of talking to me today?

In this response, I extrapolate from what Shell Annette has said about her strengths, that she is brave and can do things, before asking for her goal.

Shell Annette: … I think the fact that I've put myself out there… I think I'd feel quite good in myself, that I've actually been brave enough to do that.

Windy: So, if we stopped the session right now, you would have achieved what you aimed to do.

Shell Annette: Yes.

The client makes the point that she has already achieved her goal.

Windy: So, anything else is a bonus.

Shell Annette: Yes.

Windy: Let's give you a bonus. What kinds of things do you make yourself anxious about?

Shell Annette: … I'm very busy. I'm a really hard worker. I have a lot to do. And I think I've realised I've used it over the years as an avoidance. If I keep myself so busy, I don't have to think about my life, about me, if I just keep myself on the go all the time.

Windy: Right. So, when you realised that you were doing that, did that lead to any change?

Shell Annette: Yeah. I suppose it calmed me down quite a lot in sometimes being able to relax and think, 'Shell Annette, just give yourself a little bit of time.' But I always seem to slip back into it and just have lots of things to do.

Windy: What kinds of things are we talking about?

Shell Annette: Well, I've got my own business, so every year I've got my accounts to do, which is now – stock-taking. I'm doing a degree at the minute, so I'm busy with that. I've got a horse. I've got my dogs. Even when I go now and ride my horse, there are some days that I think, 'Do you know, I'm not going to take my phone today,' or, 'I'm going to take my watch off,' and that's the time I can truly relax.

Windy: You do that, do you?

Shell Annette: I do, yeah, at times. I've just only recently.

Windy: So, there are times when you choose, decide to not take your watch with you and to not take your phone with you.

Shell Annette: Yeah.

Windy: And, at those times, you relax.

Shell Annette: Yes.

Windy: OK. And you've just made that decision?

Shell Annette: Just recently, yeah, not too long ago.

Windy: Yeah, OK. Is that something that you see that you could do more of?

This is an example of how to capitalise on helpful strategies the client has used in the past to deal with her anxiety.

Shell Annette: [Pause] Well, yeah, but probably just not at the minute because I'm also in the middle of converting my shop into a flat, so I'm having to arrange everything for that. And, I suppose, what I'm really thinking is just, 'Thank God

I'm finishing this course in May, and I'm finished then,' and then I feel that I'll have more time, come May.

Windy: Right.

Shell Annette: But then, knowing me, I'll fill it with something else.

Windy: Right. So, if you weren't filling all your time up, what would you have to come face to face with?

Shell Annette: [Pause] I suppose I'd have to come face to face first with me, but then, having said that, I have looked at myself a lot over the past couple of years or few years.

Windy: So, you've looked at yourself a lot.

Shell Annette: Yeah.

Windy: And you were saying that you've had to come face to face with yourself, and you've looked at yourself a lot, and what's the conclusion?

Shell Annette: … I think the big thing is… through personal counselling, it's building up my self-worth, which I have been doing because I have very low self-worth. To build that up, I feel a lot better. I'm actually happy in my own company. I can be on my own. But then I think I go to extremes of probably isolating myself from people as well.

Windy: So, you can go to both extremes: you can isolate yourself, and you can do the busyness.

Shell Annette: Yeah.

Windy: So, what would be the ideal balance for you?

I am having some difficulty getting a stable goal from Shell Annette. Here I try again.

Shell Annette: … Somewhere in the middle… where… [Pause] Do you know, this question I asked the other day – do you know what I'd love to do? I would just love to sit and watch a film, and I just think, God, that would just be so relaxing, because, as I say, I don't have time to watch TV.

Shell Annette comes up with a specific activity that embodies her goal.

Windy: Can I just clarify something, in terms of what you mean? Are you saying you don't have time to watch TV or you don't make time to watch TV?

Shell Annette: [Pause] I probably don't make time to watch TV.

Windy: Does that feel different to say that?

Shell Annette: It does, yes.

Windy: In what way?

Shell Annette: [Pause] Because I think, if I always think, 'Oh, I've got this to do, I've got that to do, I've got the other to do,' I put myself under pressure: 'I've got to do this, I've got to do that, I've got to do the other,' when it feels great, in fact, if I was to think, 'Do you know, actually, why don't you make that hour or two hours to do that?' That would really relax me.

Having helped Shell Annette to see that there is a difference between 'making time,' which involves an active choice, and 'having time,' which does not and which leads Shell Annette to rehearse a number of rigid ideas, I return to the specific goal.

Windy: Right, OK. And do you have any particular film that you'd like to watch?

Shell Annette: Any kids' film. I love kids' films.

Windy: Any kids' film. Do you have a TV?

Shell Annette: I do, yeah.

Windy: Do you have satellite TV?

Shell Annette: Yeah.

Windy: Sky Disney channel or something?

Shell Annette: Well, I've just bought a new television, and it's got Netflix on. So, I could actually go onto that.

Windy: OK. When would you like to do that?

Having ascertained that Shell Annette has agreed to watch a kids' film on Netflix, I ask her to specify a time when she will do this.

Shell Annette: When?

Windy: Yeah.

Shell Annette: [Pause] I'd like to do it now, tonight.

Windy: OK. What time?

Shell Annette: … 7 o'clock.

Windy: 7 o'clock, OK. So, let's see if we can introduce a bit of realism here. At ten to seven you start thinking, 'I haven't got time for this, because I have to do that, I have to do this, I have to do that, I have to do that.' Let's suppose that happens, right? How are you going to respond to that part of yourself?

Having agreed a goal with Shell Annette, I ask her to imagine an obstacle to achieving it that she mentioned earlier and how she would address it.

Shell Annette: I'm going to say, 'Make time. Make that time for you.'

Windy: Yeah. And I might suggest that you say, 'Actually, no I don't have to do that.'

Shell Annette: Yeah.

Windy: It's a choice.

Here I suggest that Shell Annette responds to her 'have tos' and use the concept of 'choice' discussed earlier.

Shell Annette: Yeah.

Windy: It's not a 'have to'.

Shell Annette: Yeah.

Windy: OK? So, maybe, if you kind of think in terms of, rather than 'have tos', you think in terms of choices, because when you get into the zone of choice, if you like, or the land of choice, I think I even had the sense when you were doing that, you found that a bit more relaxing, as opposed to, 'I have to do this, I have to do that', as opposed to, 'No, I don't. I can choose.'

Shell Annette: Yeah.

Windy: Which one is associated with anxiety and which one is associated with calming down a bit, do you think?

Shell Annette: Well, it's me putting myself under pressure, isn't it? It's me thinking 'I have to, I have to.'

Windy: Yeah. And, if you say, 'No, I don't, I can choose to,' how do you feel?

Shell Annette: That makes it so much easier and so much calmer.

Windy: So, can you see the relationship between your anxiety and, on the one hand, all these 'have tos' that you're initially coming up with?

Shell Annette: Yeah.

Here, I ask Shell Annette to reflect on the connections between her rigid and flexible basic attitudes and her unhealthy and healthy negative emotions (Dryden, 2016). I am using this framework here in response to what Shell Annette has said during the course of the session, beginning at the outset.

Windy: By the way, it's a bit like what I was saying to Steve – that will be your default position but, just like on a computer, just because something defaults to something, it doesn't mean that you have to go along with it.

Steve was the first client I saw that day.

Shell Annette: Yeah.

Windy: You can choose to change it.

Shell Annette: Yeah.

Windy: So, I just wanted to be realistic; that you may well find yourself with those shoulds, but you say, 'Uh-uh, no, wait a minute, no, I don't have to. I have a choice.'

Shell Annette: Yeah.

Windy: OK. So, if you go home at ten to seven and part of you says, 'No, I don't have time for this because I should be doing that,' you can say, 'No, I don't have to. I have a choice.' Can you imagine doing that?

Shell Annette: Yeah, I can imagine doing that.

Windy: OK, good. Where would you be?

Shell Annette: Sorry?

Windy: Where would you be in your house doing that? Which room?

Shell Annette: In the living room.

Windy: Yeah? So, can you see yourself initially starting to have those shoulds and then being aware of that and saying, 'No, no. I don't have to. I have a choice. I can choose to make time for myself right now and sit down and watch TV'?

Shell Annette: Yeah.

Windy: Can you imagine yourself doing that?

Shell Annette: I can see myself doing that.

Windy: And how do you feel when you do that?

Shell Annette: I feel a lot better, a lot calmer.

Here I use imagery to encourage Shell Annette to rehearse the solution in the session.

Windy: OK. So, again, I think that when you have started to look at yourself and started doing some of the work that you've mentioned, that you've started to develop a sense of self-worth, self-esteem. You've actually seen the benefits of what happens when you can choose to make time by taking your watch off, and you can choose to make time by not taking your phone, and you can choose to make time to sit down and watch a film. Now, do you have any fear about what would happen if you did more of this and became more focused on your own development, your own relaxation? Do you have any fears about what would happen in your life if you do that?

Shell Annette: What? If I was to take more time for me?

Windy: Yeah. Is there a downside for you?

Shell Annette: The downside is, would I get everything done that I have to do? That would be the downside. But the upside would be, it would be absolutely great for me.

Windy: OK. So, the downside is, 'Would I get everything done that I have to do?'

Shell Annette: Yeah.

Windy: OK. Well, let's just see. Are you breathing at the moment?

At this point my intention is to help Shell Annette see that she has only a few 'needs' – things she has to have or she will die – but I don't explain what I am doing or make the most of this intervention.

Shell Annette: Yes.

Windy: OK. That's good because you have to do that, don't you, because otherwise, if you don't do that, what?

Shell Annette: I'll die.

Windy: OK, so you're doing that?

Shell Annette: Yes.

Windy: OK. Do you drink water?

Shell Annette: No, not very often.

Windy: Well, you drink?

Shell Annette: I drink coffee.

Windy: OK, well, that contains water, and you know you have to do that. Do you know why?

Shell Annette: To keep me hydrated.

Windy: Yeah, because if you don't do that, what?

Shell Annette: I'll die.

Windy: OK. So, that's two needs you're doing. So, what other needs do you have to do?

Shell Annette: [Pause] Look after myself.

Windy: OK, right, you can say that, but you didn't have that in mind when I asked you about the fear. When you said, 'I may not be able to do everything I have to do,' you didn't have looking after yourself in mind, did you?

Shell Annette: No.

Windy: What did you have in mind?

Shell Annette: That I wouldn't have time to do it.

Windy: What? That's what I'm saying. What wouldn't you have the time to do, because you've got the time to drink water, you've got the time to breathe, you've got time to look after yourself? What other 'have tos' do you not have time for?

Shell Annette: What do you mean? Like work?

Windy: I don't know.

Shell Annette: Yeah, work and getting everything organised for downstairs, to get it in on time when people are coming in to work, like the plumber, the electrician, getting everything on time for them.

Windy: And are they dictating their time to you or are you dictating the time to them?

Shell Annette: A bit of both.

Windy: OK. What would happen if you took more in charge with these tradesmen, if you were in charge more?

Shell Annette: Well, that would help if I was in charge, but I've got to go along with them, when they can actually fit in to do the job.

Windy: OK, alright. But what would happen if you don't manage to fit in with them?

Shell Annette: Well, they wouldn't be able to come and do the job that day.

Windy: And therefore?

Shell Annette: It would put it back for another day.

Windy: Yeah, and if it was put back another day, how bad would that be for you?

Shell Annette: I was just going to say I'd die, but I wouldn't really, would I?

While my 'needs' intervention fizzles out, Shell Annette does come to see that not having her so-called 'needs' met will not be a life-and-death matter. As will be seen below, she resonates with this idea.

Windy: Right. Well, I don't know. We could do the experiment, but do you see what I'm saying? It's almost like you're reacting as if terrible things will happen.

Shell Annette: I know, yeah.

Windy: As opposed to things being inconvenient, you see?

Shell Annette: Yeah.

Windy: So, what do you think would happen if you stopped looking at things as life and death, and started looking at things as either inconvenient or convenient?

Here, I show Shell Annette that she can generalise this solution.

Shell Annette: Yeah.

Windy: Right?

Shell Annette: Yeah, you've really hit it on the head there.

Windy: Yeah?

Shell Annette: Yeah.

Windy: OK. So, why don't you summarise what you're going to take away today?

Shell Annette's response indicates that she resonates with the idea of seeing things as convenient or inconvenient, as opposed to life or death. As we are nearing the end of the session, I use this as an opportunity to ask her to summarise the whole session.

Shell Annette: I'm going to take away the urgency to have to do things – the language. Giving myself more time and knowing I have the choices to do that.

Windy: And to start seeing things as inconveniences rather than life or death matters.

Shell Annette: Yeah.

Windy: But I would recommend that you keep drinking liquids and keep breathing.

Shell Annette: Yeah.

Windy: I think that's important.

I end the session on a light-hearted note, which helps to bring about closure.

Shell Annette: Yeah, I'll do that.

Windy: Right. Are we done?

Shell Annette: … Yeah.

Windy: Are you happy?

Shell Annette: Yeah.

Windy: Good. OK, let's see what they have to say.

Shell Annette: Thank you.

I invite the audience to ask me or Shell Annette questions or make observations.

General comments on the session

I think that the above session demonstrates the following elements of my approach.

Strengths-based emphasis

From the outset, I was looking to identify and help Shell Annette use her strengths. I highlighted the fact that Shell Annette was acting bravely by volunteering for the interview with me, even though she felt anxious. I also took her phrase, 'I can do things' and emphasised it as a maxim of competence rather than incompetence for the session. These features show strengths-based SSC in action.

Previous helpful strategies in addressing the problem

I was vigilant to anything Shell Annette did in the past that would help her with her current problem. These were taking her watch off and leaving her phone behind. These actions helped her calm down and switch off from her 'have to'-based behavioural regime.

Goal-setting

While Shell Annette was clear at the outset that anxiety was a problem for her, I initially struggled to help her set a goal.

Eventually, she said that she wanted to achieve a balance between being busy and isolating herself and that this would be embodied by her taking time to watch a film – an activity that was *for her* in the same way that volunteering for the session was *for her*.

Focus on the client as active chooser or at the mercy of 'have tos'

This dynamic of active chooser versus slave to her 'have tos' was a major theme in the interview and is a key part of REBT theory. I helped Shell Annette to see that she had a choice in many areas where she thought she didn't. Thus, on the issue of time, she could choose to view 'time' as something that she had none of or as something that she could make for herself. She could choose to see workmen not meeting her schedule as a life-or-death matter, or she could see it as an inconvenience. Given that her goal was to live a life less dominated by anxiety, she was able to see the role that 'have tos' and 'life and death' evaluations played in her anxiety and that, if she saw life as a matter of choices and inconveniences, she could achieve her goal.

Using imagery to rehearse the solution

As shown earlier in this article, it is a feature of SSC that the counsellor encourages the client to rehearse the solution, and I did this here by encouraging Shell Annette to use imagery to rehearse sitting down and watching a film on TV, which embodied making time for herself and calming down as a result.

Anticipating and dealing with obstacles: preparing to deal with the 'have tos'

It is an important part of SSC that the counsellor helps the client to anticipate and deal with potential obstacles to pursuing their goal. In helping Shell Annette take a step towards meeting her goal by watching a film on the TV at an agreed time, I also encouraged her to consider the possibility that, just before sitting down to watch the TV film, she would think that she did not have time for this because she had to do 'x' or 'y', and if this happened, how she could deal with it.

Dealing with doubts, reservations and objections (DROs)

It is common for a client to have a doubt, reservation or objection to their agreed solution or some other part of the SSC process. In the session, Shell Annette expressed the fear that, if she focused more on her development, she would not get everything done that she 'had to' do. There followed a discussion where I encouraged her to list her needs but, in retrospect, this intervention was too open-ended, and I don't think she fully grasped the point that I was trying to make. My point was that we have fewer needs than we think we have and we have to devote time to meeting those needs that we do have. So, if looking after herself more is a 'need' for Shell Annette, then she has to devote time to this. However, I could have done this better.

Asking the client to summarise

In SSC, it is important for the client to take away what they consider to be valuable points of learning from the session. It is thus good practice for the counsellor to ask the client to summarise the session as it draws to a close, rather than summarising what transpired in the session for the client. I therefore encouraged Shell Annette to provide her own summary. In doing so, she emphasised removing the urgency of 'having to' do things, giving herself more time and knowing that she has the choice of doing so. Will she implement these 'take-aways'? It is in the nature of a demonstration of SSC in a workshop setting that I will never know, and neither will you!

In the next chapter, I will discuss whether or not clients should be followed up in SSC, and if so, how should this be done.

Reference

Dryden W (2016). *Attitudes in Rational Emotive Behaviour Therapy: components, characteristics and adversity-related consequences.* London: Rationality Publications.

Chapter 14
Follow-up in single-session counselling

Overview

There are different perspectives within the SSC community on whether clients should be followed up or not. I will review these perspectives before arguing that they should be followed up. In taking this stance, I discuss how this might be done.

To follow up or not to follow up?

Some people in the SSC community consider SSC to be what might be referred to as 'one-shot' therapy.

For these people, the central power of SSC is in the fact that it is a single session and both the counsellor and client know this at the outset. To have a pre-session contact and follow-up would, for such people, constitute an unnecessary watering down of this central power. So, for advocates of strictly 'one-shot' SSC, there would be no follow-up. However, one-shot therapy does not necessarily preclude follow-up. Although people who use walk-in single-session services may only come once, there is nothing to say that they cannot be asked if they would consent to be followed up. The same is true with the demonstrations that I do in my workshops (see Dryden, 2018). I generally don't routinely follow up with my volunteer clients, but I could, and having written this, I may well do so in the future.

The majority of people in the SSC community hold the view that SSC does not preclude further help being available and believe that SSC can be enhanced by both pre-session contact and follow-up. So what are the reasons to follow up clients who have had SSC?

Why follow up?

A follow-up session provides a variety of opportunities:

1. It provides the client with an opportunity to feedback on what they have done in the time between the face-to-face session and the follow-up session. Given that they may have formed a connection with the counsellor, they might want the person to know what happened after the session.

2. It provides the client with an opportunity to request more help if needed. Although the counsellor may have made and reiterated the point that the client can access further help at any time, having a formal follow-up may permit the client to make this request, if necessary.

3. It provides the counsellor with outcome evaluation data (ie. how the client has done). This can help the therapist improve their delivery of SST.

4. It provides the service in which the counsellor works with service evaluation data (what the client thought of the help provided). Such data can help the organisation to improve its SSC service.

When to follow up

If the counsellor and the service in which they work (if relevant) have decided to follow up clients, then the question arises, when is the best time to do so? Given that follow-up tends to occur when the client has not asked for more help after the single session, the follow-up session can be organised for the counsellor's benefit: for example, to answer a specific question, for the client's benefit or for the organisation's benefit.

- **Follow-up for the counsellor's benefit.** If the counsellor is interested in the short-term effects of the session on the client, then the follow-up session needs to be organised two or three weeks after the face-to-face session. If the counsellor is more interested in the longer-term effects of SSC, then the follow-up session can be arranged about three months after the session.
- **Follow-up for the client's benefit.** If the follow up is for the client's benefit, the counsellor should first ask the client if they would like to be followed-up. If so, they should be asked to specify the time period that suits them best.
- **Follow-up for the organisation's benefit.** When follow-up is for the organisation's benefit, it is usually because they have to justify the effectiveness of the SSC service to maintain funding. If so, then the organisation will specify the follow-up period.

My approach to follow-up

As an example of the use of follow-up in SSC, let me outline my approach to this (Dryden, 2017). At the end of the face-to-face session, I make a specific arrangement for a follow-up phone call, which lasts 20-30 minutes. I suggest that this session takes place three months after the face-to-face session, to enable any changes the client has made to mature and be incorporated into their life. As with the pre-session contact, I stress that the session needs to be scheduled at a time and place where the client can talk without distraction or interruption. I want the client to give me their full attention. Below is the framework I use in the follow-up session.

Outcome

I first enquire about matters to do with the outcome of the session:

- I begin by stating the reason why the client came for help originally.

- I ask whether the issue has changed (for better or worse) or if there has been no change.

- I ask what brought about the change, or what made the problem stay the same.

- I ask if others have noticed any change. If so, what have they noticed?

- I ask whether other areas of their life have changed for better or worse.

The session

I then ask about the client's experience of the session itself:

- What do they recall from the single session they had?

- What was particularly helpful or unhelpful?

- What use did they make of the session recording and transcript?[1]

- How satisfied are they with the counselling that they received?

- Did they find the single session to be sufficient? If not, would they wish to resume counselling? If so, would they like to see another counsellor?

- If they had any recommendations for improvement in the service that they received, what would they be?

I then ask an open question:

- 'Is there anything else I have not specifically asked you that you would like me to know?'

In the next chapter, I will examine and discuss the doubts, reservations and objections that counsellors have about SSC.

---

1. In my private SSC practice, I offer my client both a digital recording and a transcript of the session if they want it.

References

Dryden W (2018). *Very Brief Therapeutic Conversations.* Abingdon: Routledge.

Dryden W (2017). *Single-Session Integrated CBT (SSI-CBT): distinctive features.* Abingdon: Routledge.

Chapter 15
Counsellors' doubts, reservations and objections about single-session counselling

Overview

In this chapter, I will discuss the most common doubts, reservations and objections (DROs) that counsellors have about SSC. These are the ones that they express whenever I give a workshop on SSC, and my responses below reflect how I usually respond. Unless they express these DROs and enter a dialogue with someone like me about the issues involved, they will not change their views and will be unlikely to want to practise SSC. However, when they do express their DROs and engage with me in an open-minded conversation, there is a good chance that they will change their views and see the value of SSC as working best alongside other modes of counselling delivery.

'SSC is not counselling'

A common DRO that counsellors have concerning SSC is that it is not counselling. These counsellors view counselling as a professional activity that occurs over time and not in one session. They argue that the development of a counselling relationship takes time and cannot be achieved in a single session.

These views are problematic for two main reasons: first, many people only attend one session of counselling (Brown & Jones, 2005); second, it is possible to form a good working alliance in SSC (Simon et al, 2012).

One way of determining whether SSC is counselling is to consider it against the British Association for Counselling and Psychotherapy's (BACP) definition of counselling. BACP defines counselling and psychotherapy as: '... umbrella terms that cover a range of talking therapies. Counsellors and psychotherapists are trained professionals who will work with you over a period of time to help you develop a better understanding of yourself and of others. Therapists are impartial. They will listen to you without judgement and work with your emotions without becoming emotional themselves. They won't tell you what to do but will help you find your own solutions – whether for making effective changes or for learning how to cope.'[1]

Note that BACP does not define the 'period of time' and, as SSC is designed to help the client 'develop a better understanding of yourself and of others... [and] help you find your own solutions', I would argue it is counselling by BACP's definition.

'Real change happens slowly and gradually'

Different clients probably want different things from counselling. While some clients may want 'real change', whatever that means, others seem to want SSC, and of those, 70–80% of clients are satisfied with that single session, given their current circumstances (Hoyt & Talmon, 2014a). Why should counsellors discredit what a sizeable proportion of clients say they find helpful by denying that it is counselling? In my view, this view is not tenable.

1.www.bacp.co.uk/media/8274/bacp-introduction-counselling-psychotherapy-client-information-sheet-april-2020.pdf (accessed 22 May 2020).

'Effective counselling is built on the therapeutic relationship, which takes time to develop'

Effective counselling of *varying lengths* is founded on the therapeutic relationship (Norcross & Lambert, 2019).[2] The important term here is 'varying lengths'. As already mentioned, it does seem that a good outcome in SSC is associated with the development of a good working alliance between counsellor and client in that session (Simon et al, 2012). So, effective practitioners can develop a good therapeutic relationship with clients in SSC, which, in my view, counters the above objection.

'Relational depth cannot be achieved in SSC'

Mearns and Cooper (2018: xxvii) describe relational depth in counselling as:

> ... a state of profound contact and engagement between two people, in which each person is fully real with the Other, and able to understand and value the Other's experiences at a high level.

There is no doubt that, for many clients who stay in counselling for long enough, meeting their counsellors at relational depth can be profoundly therapeutic, and it may well be the case that most counsellors in SSC do not achieve such a deep relationship with most of their clients. However, as noted above, different clients want different things from counselling, and many other clients do not seem to want or need this kind of counselling relationship. As such, this viewpoint is best seen as an observation rather than a DRO.

'SSC is a quick fix'

In Chapter 4, I discussed the goals of SSC. There I said that the SSC practitioner aims to help the client a) to get unstuck by encouraging them to find a solution to their problem, and b) to

---

2. In this book, I use the terms 'therapeutic relationship', 'counselling relationship' and 'working alliance' synonymously.

develop an action plan to implement this solution, which will lead them to take a few steps forward. Often, for many people, this forward momentum is all they need to take up the reins of change for themselves.

The online Cambridge Dictionary defines a 'quick fix' as 'something that seems to be a fast and easy solution to a problem but is in fact not very good or will not last long'. As can be seen from this definition, there are two elements to a 'quick fix': a) an easily found solution, and b) a solution that lacks durability. SSC aims to help the client find the first but not the second. Also, the concept of a quick fix ignores the process nature of SSC. A major goal of SSC is to help the client find something that they can take forward and use in the future. It is unrealistic to expect the client's problem to be fixed at the end of the session, but quite realistic to expect that they will find a solution that they can implement going forward.

'SSC is a sticking-plaster solution'

Counsellors sometimes say that SSC offers a sticking plaster solution. The online Cambridge Dictionary defines a 'sticking plaster' in this context as 'dealing with a problem in a temporary and unsatisfactory way'. Factually, a sticking plaster is put on a wound to protect it, keep it clean and aid healing. So, I would agree that SSC provides a sticking plaster solution in that it aids healing, but not that it does so in a temporary and unsatisfactory way. When the counsellor and client search for solutions in the session, they are looking for one that the client can implement to aid long-term healing, not one that provides temporary relief but will not solve the client's problem.

'SSC means that people will not get what they need therapeutically'

This view is centred on the question, 'Who decides what a client needs therapeutically?' If the therapist determines the client's need, then they will assess the client and carry out a case formulation and a case history. From this approach, the therapist is likely to form a view concerning what problems the client has and what they need therapeutically in terms of 'treatment' for these problems. This will usually involve the offer of a block of counselling sessions, which the client will have to wait for if the agency is in the public or non-profit sector.

If the client determines their own need, then they get to have a say in how to go forward. If they want to be assessed and then be offered treatment based on that assessment, and if they are prepared to wait for both the initial assessment and the subsequent treatment, then they should be able to do this. However, if they want to have a single session of counselling with a minimal wait, to see if they can get meaningful help for their prioritised problem from that session, knowing that further help may be available, then they should be able to do this too.

If they choose the latter option, then they are getting what they need therapeutically because they have determined that need.

'People in charge of funding push SSC because it saves money'

Counsellors sometimes take the view that SSC is being encouraged mainly because it saves money, and this DRO may well be justified. However, this should not be the main reason for introducing it in a counselling agency. SSC should ideally be introduced because it provides help at the point of need rather than at the point of availability. If it also saves money, so much the better, but this should be the by-product of its introduction, not the prime reason for its introduction.

'SSC means one session and one session only'

Some counsellors have DROs about SSC because they think that it means one session and one session only. As I discussed in Chapter 1, there may be times when clients are only offered one session in SSC. However, most commonly SSC is seen as a session where counsellor and client set out with the intention of helping the client in that session with the knowledge that more help is available. As such, when SSC is one session only, it is that way mainly because the client has decided to have only one session and not because the client wants more help and this is being refused by the counsellor or by the agency in which the counsellor works.

'SSC is 5, 10 or more sessions "distilled" into one'

In 1953, the BBC made a film of the train journey between London Victoria and Brighton, speeded up to last for four minutes.[3] In Chapter 10, I argued that SSC has an intrinsic process and is not a distillation of a larger number of sessions. In short, SSC is not counselling 'at speed'. Rather, it has its own process and its own rhythm, as shown in Chapters 10 and 12 and as demonstrated in Chapter 13.

'SSC is only appropriate for simple problems'

Quite a common criticism of SSC is that it is only appropriate for people who have simple problems. This view is at odds with the experiences of those who offer SSC in different contexts and different countries around the world. It is also not borne out by research that shows that people with complex problems can and have been helped by SSC (see Hoyt & Talmon, 2014a).

'SSC is not for vulnerable clients'

Clients who are vulnerable need help when that vulnerability has been activated. SSC provides them with an opportunity to access such help when they need it. When I give SSC training workshops for university counselling services, a major concern is how to respond to a student at risk in SSC. As discussed in Chapter 12, my reply is that the counsellor responds to them in the same way as they would in another counselling context, with one difference: the counsellor gets to find about this risk sooner in SSC than in these other counselling contexts. Also, vulnerable clients are not always vulnerable and may still have

---

3. See www.youtube.com/watch?v=TtiWQkW0v0o (accessed 22 August 2019).

problems for which they can be seen safely in SSC. Thus, a client with borderline personality disorder may be anxious about an imminent job interview for which they would like prompt help.

'SSC means a restriction on counselling sessions'

In Chapter 1, I discussed a concept known as one-at-a-time counselling (OAATC). This means that clients who require more counselling after the single session can have it, but only one session at a time, and before they can book another session, they are encouraged to reflect on and digest what they have learned, put this learning into practice and see what happens. This means that no restrictions are placed on the number of sessions a client can have. If this is compared with the usual situation where clients are offered a finite block of counselling sessions, it can be seen that it is this practice, rather than SSC/ OAATC, that restricts counselling sessions.

'SSC practitioners think that SSC is the answer to everything'

This criticism has very little merit, in my view. There is nothing in the published SSC literature to indicate that people in the SSC community think that 'SSC is the answer to everything' (eg. Hoyt & Talmon, 2014b; Hoyt et al, 2018). Rather, SSC is portrayed in these publications as a timely response to client need in a variety of contexts, but only for those people who wish to take advantage of it.

'SSC practitioners think that SSC is for everyone'

Again, this is not the case. SSC practitioners hold that SSC is only for people who make an informed decision to have it, and therefore it should not be imposed on people who do not want it. Also, SSC is not for all counsellors. For example, there are some counsellors who hold that they can't practise SSC – for example, because they can't offer counselling without first conducting a case history or a case formulation. Also, some counsellors do not agree with the SSC mindset and so do not wish to practise it. Their decision should be respected.

'SSC is the same as crisis intervention'

When they first encounter SSC, some counsellors see it as the same as crisis intervention. While SSC can be practised with clients in crisis (Hoyt & Talmon, 2014b), it is not synonymous with crisis intervention. SSC practitioners can and do work with a range of clients who need help but are not in crisis (Hoyt et al, 2018).

'SSC is simpler than longer-term therapy because it is brief and focused'

A commonly expressed view about SSC is that it is simpler to practise than longer-term therapy because it is brief and focused. An alternative viewpoint is that it is harder to practise than longer-term therapy because the counsellor needs to use a variety of skills in a very short time period. In my opinion, there is no definitively correct position on this point and both modes of counselling delivery have their complexities. As such, this DRO should not be a reason for a counsellor to dismiss SSC out of hand.

In the final chapter, I consider what research says about SSC.

References

Brown GS, Jones ER (2005). Implementation of a feedback system in a managed care environment: what are patients teaching us? *Journal of Clinical Psychology 61*: 187–198.

Hoyt MF, Bobele M, Slive A, Young J, Talmon M (eds) (2018). *Single Session Therapy by Walk-In or Appointment: administrative, clinical, and supervisory aspects of one-at-a-time services.* New York, NY: Routledge.

Hoyt MF, Talmon MF (2014a). What the literature says: an annotated bibliography. In: Hoyt MF, Talmon M (eds). *Capturing the Moment: single session therapy and walk-in services.* Bethel, CT: Crown House Publishing (pp487–516).

Hoyt MF, Talmon M (eds) (2014b). *Capturing the Moment: single session therapy and walk-in services.* Bethel, CT: Crown House Publishing.

Mearns D, Cooper M (2018). *Working at Relational Depth in Counselling and Psychotherapy* (2nd ed). London: Sage.

Norcross JC, Lambert MJ (eds) (2019). *Psychotherapy Relationships that Work. Volume 1: evidence-based therapist contributions.* New York, NY: Oxford University Press.

Simon GE, Imel ZE, Ludman EJ, Steinfeld BJ (2012). Is dropout after a first psychotherapy visit always a bad outcome? *Psychiatric Services, 63*(7): 705–707.

Chapter 16
Is single-session counselling effective?

In preparing this chapter reviewing the effectiveness of SSC, I did an initial search on 'single session-counselling' on the PsycINFO electronic database, which returned 86 results. However, given that investigations of the effectiveness of single-session approaches have also used or drawn on terms such as 'single-session therapy' (eg. Hoyt & Talmon, 2014a), 'single-session psychotherapy' (eg. Bloom, 2001) and 'walk-in single sessions' (eg. Slive et al, 1995), I broadened my literature search to include these and similar terms (and I will use all three terms interchangeably in this review). Widening the search also identified a far greater number of sources that could have relevance to this chapter's title. For example, a search for 'single-session therapy' returned 326 results, of which 202 were journal articles, 93 were books (mainly book chapters), 27 were dissertations and four were electronic collections.

Having considered that there are different types and a large number of potential sources that relate to the effectiveness of SSC, I will go on to examine examples of these sources, and how several authors have reviewed them to evaluate the effectiveness of single-session counselling.

Aafjes-van Doorn and Sweeney (2019) have noted that typical reviews of single-session treatments can be broken down into narrative and systematic reviews. Narrative reviews typically consider a number of author-selected case studies (or 'clinical overviews and program descriptions' (Bloom, 2001)) that assume SSC is effective and research/outcome studies relating to the SSC field in general (eg. Bloom, 2001; Campbell, 2012; Hurn, 2005) and, in one case, walk-in psychotherapy (Cameron, 2007). Systematic reviews are based on a comprehensive search of research studies relating to the effectiveness of SSC, from which studies are selected on the basis of explicit exclusion and inclusion criteria (eg. criteria relating to the study participants/patients, presenting problems, purpose of the review, the type of SST provided, study design, study context etc). In discussing research studies, the narrative reviews tend to describe studies and (usually) provide some methodological considerations, whereas the systematic reviews provide more structured reporting of studies – for example, to aid comparisons – and they usually go into more critical (and sometimes systematic) detail regarding the methodological quality of studies. The discussion below will discuss narrative and systematic reviews in turn.

Narrative reviews – case studies

As part of a review of the clinical and research literature relating to focused single-session psychotherapy, Bloom (2001) refers to a clinical chapter by Rosenbaum, Hoyt and Talmon (1990), 'The challenge of single-session therapies: creating pivotal moments'. In this chapter, the authors note that, in their psychiatric clinic, 'approximately 30% of our clients are seen for only a single session, despite having prepaid coverage entitling them to additional sessions if indicated' (p166). However, they also observe that many therapists 'have difficulties accepting the fact that change can occur in a single session' (p167). They associate this with several 'therapist resistances to brief therapy in general', which can be characterised by beliefs such as 'more is better' and 'for therapy to be effective, "deep" character changes must be accomplished' (p167). They discuss the erroneous nature of such beliefs and barriers in the light of literature that suggests

(Ticho, 1972) that 'SSTs and other brief therapies provide what is needed when it is needed' (p169) and that client resistance can be reduced or effectively managed in a single session. Rosenbaum and colleagues then focus on how to plan for, and carry out, intentional SST effectively, with reference to effective case-study illustrations. In so doing, they discuss 'recognising when a patient may benefit from SST' (for example, by considering the patient's motivation and expectations of therapy duration, and the success of previously attempted solutions) (p169), and 'basic heuristic and technical principles for SST', including specific helpful therapist attitudes for promoting single-session therapies (such as to 'expect change' and to 'view each encounter as a whole') (pp171–175).

Rosenbaum, Hoyt and Talmon's (1990) discussion above concerns 'issues involved in planning for and successfully conduction of intentional single-session therapies' (p166) in general. In addition, Bloom (2001: 78) has noted that 'specific theoretical orientations to single-session psychotherapy have been described'. For example, he refers (p79) to an examination of 'the usefulness of *Gestalt theory* and techniques in the context of single-session psychotherapy' (Harman, 1995) and an article by Albert Ellis (1989) on the use of a single session of rational-emotive therapy (RET) when working with a suicidal woman.

In the latter article, Ellis notes the overlap of RET and Adlerian individual psychology in that, for example, 'it is active-directive and problem-solving' and 'it briefly and authoritatively zeroes in on clients' basic irrational beliefs and mistaken life-styles and helps them subsequently to do this for themselves' (p75). Ellis states that 'RET is useful in crisis intervention just because, as Adler advocated, it quickly gets to the core philosophies that tend to drive people to states of panic, depression and suicidalness' (p76). Ellis discusses how he took a highly encouraging attitude toward the suicidal client, and also outlines three techniques that he used and that are useful in this kind of crisis intervention: 'the therapist giving the client unconditional acceptance,' 'refusal to be intimidated by the client's strong suicidal leanings' and 'the active-directive approach of showing suicidal clients how life can be a fascinating challenge rather than an empty bore' (p80). He later received feedback that the client had completely given up her suicidal ideas after her one session with him.[1]

In addition to discussing the clinical literature on SSC in general and with reference to specific theoretical orientations, Bloom (2001) notes (pp79–80) that single-session psychotherapy has been reported as being particularly useful in the treatment of medical disorders, such as group work with cancer patients in an acute-care hospital (Block, 1985), and for physicians working with families who face medical dilemmas (Erstling & Devlin, 1989); in the treatment of drug addiction, such as crack cocaine addiction (Marcus, 1999) and problem drinking (Miller, 2000); in the treatment of adolescents (Slaff, 1995) and college students in public schools and university settings (Cooper & Archer, 1999), and when dealing with interpersonal conflicts, including family or marital stress (Brown, 1984).

Bloom also outlines a study relating to a walk-in counselling service in Calgary, Canada (Slive et al, 1995), in which client families gain immediate access to systemically trained therapists at times that the families choose. The authors of this study describe this as an 'extraordinarily responsive and cost-efficient service' (Slive et al, 1995: 11). Writing somewhat later (2012), Campbell notes that the literature of SST services descriptions have been dominated by offerings from Canada, including further developments led by Slive (Slive et al, 2008). Campbell suggests that descriptions such as these provide 'considerable organisational and experiential evidence that these services work' (p23).

More recent clinical overviews and descriptions that claim to demonstrate the effectiveness of SSC or how to practise it effectively have emerged in chapters in edited books, such as

---

1. Ellis received this positive feedback from the client's regular therapist, so it could be argued that this was not strictly a SSC case study. However, it raises the possibility of considering the possible benefits of having SSC as an adjunct to regular therapy.

Hoyt and Talmon (2014a) and Hoyt et al (2018a). Programme descriptions from walk-in clinics in Canada continue to have some prominence (as noted earlier by Campbell), as do those in Australia, and there are also interesting case studies of novel or emerging applications of SSC, such as 'Single session walk-in therapy for street robbery victims in Mexico City' (Platt & Mondellini, 2014) and 'Equine-assisted single session consultations' (Green, 2014), as well as the adaptation of single-session therapy to acute emergency settings in post-disaster Haiti (Guthrie, 2018), where 'a case example is provided to illustrate both what can be accomplished and limitations when facing major disruptions and lack of social services' (Hoyt et al, 2018b: 17).

This also encourages us to consider ways in which the effectiveness of SSC can be influenced by the context in which it occurs and related developments in this area of the clinical literature. These would include recent chapters based on many years of accumulated practice that focus on administrative, service delivery and supervisory aspects that might promote the effective practice of SSC. For example, Young, Rycroft and Weir (2014) have discussed and offer practical strategies for the implementation of SST into regular service delivery (such as improving the chances of implementation success by linking SST to existing organisational processes, procedures, policy and strategic directions, and to practitioner values and the philosophy of the host organisation). Hoyt et al (2018a) also offer three chapters relating to SST supervision, including the teaching of skills that prepare interns and new therapists for walk-in counselling (Bedggood, 2018), and group supervision that is designed to promote evidence-based practice, review and reflection by the therapist, 'and to provide the funding organization with some assurances about the quality of the services' (Harper-Jaques, 2018: 344).

In considering the case study and clinical overview literature, it is important to note that these are not systematic studies of the effectiveness of SSC, but (often) enthusiastic descriptions of SSC or SSC practice that authors claim, or assume, to be effective (albeit there are increasing examples of learning from experiential evidence and evidence-based practice). Hurn (2005: 37) has also observed 'that there are few demographic details to be had in any of these studies. Central issues like the use of previous therapy are omitted or unknown'. However, I have noted at least two examples where authors have referred to concurrent therapy – for example, Ellis (1989) and Green (2014) (where Green notes that equine therapy is as an additional experiential component to intensive therapy for couples). Hurn (2005: 37) does also note that 'case studies like these have encouraged writers to consider the many factors at play in single sessions and whether they enable the client or the therapist in promoting greater change. The subjective elements to this methodology do enable different perspectives to be aired which can inform the exploratory nature of this phenomenon. This may then lead to a more defined understanding of just what constitutes Single-Session Therapy'.

Having considered the nature of the clinical literature, and noted some of its advantages and limitations, I will now examine some of the research evidence regarding the effectiveness of SSC.

The research case for the effectiveness of SSC – narrative reviews

Hoyt and Talmon (2014b) provide examples of many research studies relating to the effectiveness of SST. These include various papers (Hoyt & Talmon, 2014b) that indicate that the most common length of therapy is one visit (p493). Interestingly, Hoyt and colleagues (2018b: 7) consider this fact (rather than effectiveness) to be the most significant evidence supporting the adoption of SST. However, Hoyt and Talmon (2014b) also reference many research papers that support its effectiveness. Such papers include those that have reported that a single session is often what is needed from a client's point of view; significant reduction of distress and problem severity and also improvements in client satisfaction after a single session; the effectiveness of a single session with problems of anxiety, alcohol and substance abuse and self-harming behaviour, and that single sessions of therapy can be associated with generalised life improvements over and above symptom relief.

Other authors have similarly examined the research into the effectiveness of SST (for example, Bloom, 2001; Hurn, 2005; Campbell, 2012; Cameron, 2007). In such papers, the authors have included reviews of selected individual outcome studies (in addition to individual case studies) – both uncontrolled and controlled. An example of an uncontrolled outcome study that is frequently discussed is Talmon (1990). This study was prompted by Talmon's coincidental discovery that unplanned SST was the most common length of therapy where he worked. In this exploratory investigation, Talmon (along with therapists Hoyt and Rosenbaum) carried out planned SST with a heterogeneous sample of 60 patients, and then carried out follow-up evaluations of these sessions. The evaluations involved a telephone interview (which followed a protocol they developed), by someone other than the therapist, three to 12 months after the session (Talmon 1990: 15). They were able to contact 58 of the sample for follow-up interview. Of those 58, 88% reported either 'much improvement' or 'improvement' since the session, 79% thought that the SST had been sufficient, and 34 (58%) reported that they did not require additional sessions (this had also been agreed with the therapist at the end of the session, and they had received no further therapy between the session and the time they were called for follow-up). However, three patients reported no improvement or felt that SST had not been sufficient.

As Bloom (2001: 80) has noted, while uncontrolled outcome studies (such as that described above) 'testify to the effectiveness of single-session psychotherapy, their design does not yield as persuasive data as would be obtained when appropriately selected comparison groups would be studied at the same time'. He therefore also considers seven controlled outcome studies (some with random assignment to treatment conditions) 'designed to provide contrasting data on single-session psychotherapy treatment outcomes and one or more other treatment modalities', and where 'similar follow-up data were collected from the various treatment groups' (pp80–81). By way of illustration, one such study (Askevold, 1983) compared the outcome of three different forms of therapy – single interview, brief psychotherapy and regular psychotherapy – among three groups of patients being treated for anorexia nervosa. The study reported no differences among the three groups with respect to selection and other criteria (such as weight loss, social background, duration of illness etc). In the follow-up, four to 14 years later, the study found no differences between the groups, although 'the regular psychotherapy group was slightly worse off than the two others, but not to a significant degree' (Askevold, 1983: 193).

Bloom (2001) concluded from his review (which included case studies, as well as outcome studies) that, while the existing literature was rather limited and of 'insufficient methodological rigor' (p75), the evidence suggested that a 'variety of theoretical perspectives are equally effective in enhancing the usefulness of a single-session treatment episode' (p83), and that 'under some as yet unspecifiable conditions, single session of psychotherapy may be broadly effective in achieving a variety of clinical goals' (Bloom, 2001: 83). He argued that additional controlled outcome research studies are needed 'to evaluate with greater confidence the conditions under which single-session psychotherapy may be particularly appropriate' (p83).

Later narrative reviews of the research also concluded that single-session psychotherapy 'can be used to address a diverse array of presenting problems and has a demonstrated ability to satisfy client expectations' (Cameron, 2007: 248) and that 'there is no harm in using a single session, and considerable evidence that, around half the time, that is all that is necessary to lead to meaningful change' (Campbell, 2012: 23).

Although these narrative reviews of the research help to illustrate SSC and provide some evidence of situations where it has been effective, they are not intended as a formal or comprehensive review of the literature. Aafjes-van Doorn and Sweeney (2019) also suggest that the validity of their conclusions is unknown, due to possible selection bias associated with 'ad hoc' choices of outcome studies (a similar point could also be made with respect to their earlier noted choices of case studies), and the limited consideration given to the methodological adequacy of the reviewed studies.

With such limitations in mind, I will now discuss systematic reviews.

The research case for the effectiveness of SSC – systematic reviews

As noted earlier, systematic reviews are based on the findings of comprehensive and systematic literature searches. For example, Hymmen, Stalker and Cait (2013) examined the empirical support for the effectiveness of SSC with 'clients and presenting problems that would typically be seen in community-based mental health or counselling agencies' (p60). In doing so, they searched specified databases (such as PsycINFO and PubMed) using specified key words (such as 'single session' and other terms such as 'walk-in' and 'one-off consultation') and used clear inclusion and exclusion criteria to identify studies that were relevant to the purpose of their review. Such criteria included the requirements to include empirical outcome data, a focus on intentional SST and on clients and presenting problems that would typically be seen in community-based mental health or counselling agencies, and the exclusion of interventions that would not normally be offered at such agencies (eg. specific interventions for narrowly defined presenting problems such as specific phobias).

Hymmen and colleagues (2013) retrieved 1106 abstracts and found that 18 journal articles and book chapters met the inclusion criteria. They then listed these according to methodology, key findings and limitations of each study and summarised the key findings according to four categories (pp66–67):

* **Single-session sufficiency** – based on the data relating to clients not returning for more sessions, Hymmen and colleagues suggested that SST had been sufficient from the clients' perspective approximately 60.9% of the time.

- **Client satisfaction** – client satisfaction with the single session was assessed in half of the studies included in the review, and the findings suggested that the majority of clients in such studies were highly satisfied with SST.

- **Helpful aspects of therapy** – many studies asked what the client considered the most helpful aspect of the single-session intervention. Common themes here included 'receiving helpful advice about the problem' (five instances); 'therapist characteristics' (three instances); and 'having the opportunity to talk about the problem and feel supported' (four instances).

- **Problem improvement** – Hymmen and colleagues noted that studies 'varied as to whether they assessed change in problems generally or focused on specific problem or symptom improvement' (p66). They also varied according to factors such as when (and how often) the improvement was measured, how the improvement was measured, and whether improvements were reported as proportions of samples that had improved or as statistically significant improvements. However, all studies reported improvements (although findings in one study were not statistically significant). For example: 'Two studies reporting the proportion of the sample that self-reported improvement in the presenting problem at follow-up ranged from 67.5% (Miller & Slive, 2004) to 78% (Boyhan, 1996)' and 'three studies reported statistically significant improvements based on a scale that quantified the clients' perceptions of the presenting problem' (Hymmen, Stalker & Cait, 2013: 66–67).

Hymmen and colleagues went on to consider whether SST might work better for some clients than others. They did so in the light of two variables (identified in the studies) that may affect individuals' and families' responses to SST – namely, 'problem severity' and 'client motivation or readiness to change'. They discussed mixed findings with respect to problem severity, and also noted that clients with some presenting issues (eg. 'high risk') were excluded from some studies, which could limit the generalisability of the findings to SST provided in walk-in clinics. They make a tentative/cautious summary here that 'some agreement exists that suicidal, homicidal and psychotic clients are not appropriate for SST, and some data suggest that SST may be most effective with highly motivated, higher functioning and less distressed clients' (2013: 69).

While the studies provide some support for the effectiveness of SST, Hymmen and colleagues (2013: 69) are clear that there is a lack of sound empirical evidence for this mode of therapy. For example, relatively few (ie. 18) studies met the inclusion criteria for their review, and 'only two of these studies used randomized controlled trials (Gawrysiak, Nicholas & Hopko, 2009; Perkins, 2006), while one study used a comparison group with random assignment (Littrell, Malia & Vanderwood, 1995)'.

Hymmen and colleagues also note (2013) that these comprised a diverse range of studies with little consistency in terms of methods or instruments used to measure outcomes and effectiveness. In the latter respect, they note that the credibility of some studies was limited by the use of non-standardised measures of effectiveness (ie. measures that lacked indicators of validity and reliability). They further question the use of therapists to collect data (which raises the possibility that clients' responses may have been influenced by a desire to please their therapist) and the use of clients to provide satisfaction data (which can be skewed if, for example, clients worry about repercussions for reporting dissatisfaction). In addition, they note that 'samples have tended to be small and quite homogenous, with little information about whether the model is appropriate to diverse populations' (p69).

A couple of years later, Pitt et al (2015) reported on another systematic review of SST in the context of its relevance to sport psychology. Along with Hymmen and colleagues (2013), they were interested in the effectiveness of SST as a method of therapy, although their research included some additional aims (eg. to provide sport psychologists with an insight into the characteristics and common features of SST that distinguish this way of working from other traditional methods). These aims contributed to the choice of some somewhat different inclusion criteria in their search: for example, in addition to outcome-focused studies, they included descriptive accounts, such as case studies and overviews.

Pitt and colleagues identified 27 appropriate studies (which included some that had also been included in the Hymmen, Stalker & Cait (2013) study) and evaluated effectiveness with reference to the studies that provided outcome measures of SST's effectiveness. Helpfully, they evaluated this according to three of the effectiveness categories that Hymmen and colleagues (2013) had previously applied: problem improvement, single session sufficiency and client satisfaction.

They similarly noted that the outcome studies examined in their paper had reported problem improvements, comparable data regarding single session sufficiency, and that client satisfaction was high. In addition to reporting comparable findings to Hymmen and colleagues about the effectiveness of SST, they shared those authors' concerns about the methodological limitations (such as lack of control conditions) of the outcome studies. They did, however (drawing on Seligman, 1995), raise the interesting point that, while highly controlled studies (which Seligman refers to as 'efficacy' studies) are considered to be the 'gold standard' for measuring whether a treatment works, 'the "effectiveness" study of how patients fare under the actual conditions of treatment in the field can yield useful and credible "empirical validation" of psychotherapy' (Hymmen et al, 2013: 966). So, while there may be a lack of research related to the efficacy of SST, it seems that the studies and systematic reviews discussed in this chapter provide important validation of its effectiveness.

A more recent systematic review that included an exploration of the effectiveness of single-session therapy is by Aafjes-van Doorn and Sweeney (2019). They investigated this in relation to general adult mental health services, and in the context of a broader review of the effectiveness of initial therapy contact – ie. '(the first) 3h or less of face-to-face psychological treatment' (2019: 1). While this context encompassed 'both the early phase of a longer therapy and one-off single session therapies', the majority of the 35 studies included in their review report on stand-alone therapies – either planned single-session interventions, or a 'two-plus-one' (2+1) model developed by Barkham and colleagues (Barkham et al, 1999).

As with previous systematic reviews, qualitative synthesis of the effectiveness results suggested 'stand-alone single session(s) in a variety of therapies are effective in reducing symptoms' (Aafjes-van Doorn & Sweeney, 2019: 11). The authors also report (p11): 'Findings of the present review support the conclusion that (the first) 3h or less of therapy can possibly be an effective intervention in itself for adults with mild to moderate mental health problems. Importantly, reported effects appeared to last over time.' However, consistent with reviews such as those discussed above, the authors' quality assessment indicated that 'the majority of reviewed studies had relatively weak overall methodologies' (p11), which limited the extent to which conclusions could be drawn. For example, in discussing the study designs, they noted that only three of the 35 studies they reviewed 'fulfilled the essential features of an efficacy study' (p3), and that study results may have been influenced by other factors (such as concurrent treatments, or therapist effects), rather than the effect of initial therapy contact.

The systematic reviews above have covered what could be loosely defined as 'general' mental health services. As Aafjes-van Doorn and Sweeney also note, systematic reviews of SST have also been carried out in some more specific areas of specialism. For example, Zlomke and Davis (2008) carried out a systematic review of one-session treatment (OST) of specific phobias and concluded that 'research generally supports OST's efficacy' (p207). Schleider and Weisz (2017) also carried out a meta-analysis of single-session interventions (SSIs) for youth psychiatric problems. They identified 50 randomised controlled trials that fulfilled their inclusion criteria, and report that these SSIs 'demonstrated a significant beneficial effect in the small-to-medium range' (p113), but that several problem sub-group differences emerged. For example, 'SSIs were most effective in decreasing anxiety and conduct problems', whereas 'SSIs targeting youth depression and eating disorders had numerically promising but nonsignificant overall effects' (p113)).

While the reviews of SSC so far have been mainly positive about its effects, a systematic review of the effectiveness of single-session psychological interventions ('debriefing') following trauma (Rose, Bisson & Wesley, 2003) concluded that: 'Some outcomes following individual [psychological debriefing] were negative (notably in the studies with the longest follow-ups...) but overall, the impact of the single-session early psychological interventions in the review when considered collectively was neutral' (p181). It should also be noted that, while the studies that Rose and colleagues considered were (11) randomised controlled trials, the authors concluded that the methodological quality of the studies 'varied widely, but was generally poor' (2003: 176). This suggests the need for caution in the interpretation of their results. It could also be argued (eg. Guthrie, 2018) that single-session psychological debriefing is a specific model of therapy, and that results such as those above therefore have limited relevance to the discussion about whether SSC is effective, given that SSC is essentially a 'delivery system' or 'mindset', rather than a specific theoretical approach (Hoyt et al, 2018b; Dryden, 2019). However, Hoyt & Talmon (2014b) have also drawn on literature from 'practitioners whose theoretical models do not necessarily intend to be one session' (p487) as examples of SSC. This points to a broader problem that Hurn (2005) raised in a review of the SST literature: ie. that 'Single Session Therapy may be very hard to define' (p35) and that there is a 'limited understanding of the factors involved in a single session and how they can be identified as a specific paradigm' (p38).

Dose-response and phase models

Having considered systematic reviews of the SSC literature, this section will conclude with consideration of the findings of research and systematic reviews exploring a related area – the dose-response and phase models of psychotherapy outcomes (eg. Howard et al, 1986; Baldwin et al, 2009). Green et al (2011) note that 'these models, based on meta-analyses of outcome studies, describe substantial improvements in early stages of psychotherapy followed by ever-decreasing improvements as therapy continues' (p24). Some authors (eg. Green et al, 2011; Bloom, 2001) have used these findings to support the basis for the single session approach, with the practice of SSC taking deliberate advantage 'of the initial period of rapid improvement by keeping episodes of therapy as short as possible while at the same time encouraging clients to return for additional brief therapeutic episodes when they are needed' (Bloom, 2001: 76). With respect to returning for therapy, it has been noted (Stacey et al, 2001) that 'follow-up has not been emphasised as a component of brief therapy', whereas clients can appreciate and value this component, which can also strengthen their capacity and sense of support, as well as assist 'in the identification of early warning signs of a new problem or the recurrence of the old one' (p186). Similarly, in considering the dose-response curve literature with respect to SSC, it is also important to bear in mind (eg. Seligman, 1995) that the curve suggests that more therapy yields more improvement. Bloom (2001) also notes that there are numerous cases 'when the psychotherapeutic episode needs to be extended or when multiple brief therapeutic episodes will be needed in order to achieve satisfactory clinical objectives' (p84).

Conclusions

While the majority of the material reviewed suggests that many clients find SSC to be effective, helpful, satisfactory and sufficient, most reviews of the research have noted methodological limitations and gaps in the SSC literature. For Hurn (2005: 33), the limitations in the literature are sufficient to suggest that there is 'no conclusive evidence that SST is better than long-term therapy or that it is preferable to other more mainstream paradigms'. Given this and other considerations (such as 'limited understanding of factors involved in a single session' and 'the many cases in which SSC may be unsuitable'), he suggests that SSC might be more appropriately positioned within a triage system 'as the framework allows for a timely intervention, assessment and the opportunity for a follow-up should this be more clinically appropriate' (p39).

However, despite the methodological limitation of studies, most authors do seem to share the view that the research has generally demonstrated that many people do benefit from SSC (eg. Hoyt et al, 2018b). Campbell (2012) further considers that the literature is moving forward and supports 'a more affirmative and assertive position in relation to establishing single-session interventions' (p23), as does the considerable organisational and experiential evidence that walk-in single session services work. In addition, Cameron (2007) sees SSC as a potentially effective and 'pragmatic approach to the provision of psychotherapeutic services' in the context of diminished resources (p480). Interestingly, when researching effectiveness from a resources perspective, Lamsal et al (2018) did not find single-session walk-in counselling (SSWIC) to be cost-effective in comparison with being on a waiting list for traditional counselling. However, they found SSWIC to be more clinically effective, and they note that the model has the potential to reduce waiting lists and eliminate no-shows. They also note methodological limitations in their study, and the need for more long-term studies to support their findings.

This is just one of many areas where authors have called for more research into SSC effectiveness. Other research priorities that have been identified include the need for more outcome studies that evaluate the conditions under which single-session psychotherapy may be particularly appropriate (Bloom, 2001), and which clients most benefit from SSC and which clients may not (Hoyt et al, 2018c). Hurn (2005: 38) also draws attention to the 'limited understanding of the factors involved in a single session and they can be identified as a specific therapeutic paradigm'. In addition, Hoyt et al (2018c) consider that future trends in SSC will include developments in areas that use modern technology (such as the internet and Skype). One would hope that the use of such service delivery mediums will increasingly be accompanied and underpinned by empirical research to guide and support them.

In this respect, I note that there is recent research that suggests, for example, that improved outcomes can be achieved from a single session of web-based intervention (chat session with an online counsellor) for problem gambling (Rodda et al, 2017). However, the authors also suggest that 'online counselling requires an additional set of technical and communication skills over and above that required for traditional therapy' (p295). By way of illustration, one of these skills is time management (given that text reduces words spoken in a session). This could be all the more critical in the context of effective single-session work online, and something to consider in future research.

Whichever aspect of SSC is being investigated, the literature also suggests the need for future research to involve 'more rigorous studies with larger sample sizes, standardized measurement tools, randomization to control or comparison groups and longer-term follow-up; more diverse participants so that its effectiveness with specific client populations and presenting problems can be adequately understood; and in-depth interviews with clients to explore the active therapeutic ingredients involved within a single-session intervention' (Hymmen, Stalker & Cait, 2013: 70).

This brings us to the end of the book. I hope that you have found it useful and that it has inspired you to offer single-session interventions to your clients. I would appreciate any feedback about this book and your experiences of applying its contents. Please email me at windy@windydryden.com

References

Aafjes-van Doorn K, Sweeney K (2019). The effectiveness of initial therapy contact: a systematic review. *Clinical Psychology Review 74*: 101786. doi: 10.1016/j.cpr.2019.101786.

Askevold F (1983). What are the helpful factors in psychotherapy for anorexia nervosa? *International Journal of Eating Disorders 2*: 193–197.

Baldwin SA, Berkeljon A, Atkins DC, Olsen JA, Nielsen SL (2009). Rates of change in naturalistic psychotherapy: contrasting dose-effect and good-enough level models of change. *Journal of Consulting & Clinical Psychology 77*: 203–211.

Barkham M, Shapiro DA, Hardy GE, Rees A (1999). Psychotherapy in two-plus-one sessions: outcomes of a randomized controlled trial of cognitive-behavioral and psychodynamic-interpersonal therapy for subsyndromal depression. *Journal of Consulting and Clinical Psychology 67*: 201–211.

Bedggood J (2018). The first time: teaching skills that prepare interns and new therapists for walk-in counselling. In: Hoyt MF, Bobele M, Slive A, Young J, Talmon M (eds). *Single-Session Therapy by Walk-In or Appointment: administrative, clinical, and supervisory aspects of one-at-a-time services.* New York, NY: Routledge (pp327–333).

Block LR (1985). On the potentiality and limits of time: the single-session group and the cancer patient. *Social Work with Groups 8*: 81–99.

Bloom BL (2001). Focused single-session psychotherapy: a review of the clinical and research literature. *Brief Treatment and Crisis Intervention 1*: 75–86.

Boyhan PA (1996). Clients' perceptions of single session consultations as an option to waiting for family therapy. *Australian & New Zealand Journal of Family Therapy 17*: 85–96.

Brown LM (1984). A single consultation assessment clinic. *British Journal of Psychiatry 145*: 558.

Cameron CL (2007). Single session and walk-in psychotherapy: a descriptive account of the literature. *Counselling & Psychotherapy Research 7*: 245–249.

Campbell A (2012). Single-session approaches to therapy: time to review. *Australian & New Zealand Journal of Family Therapy 33*: 15–26.

Cooper S, Archer J (1999). Brief therapy in college counseling and mental health. *Journal of American College Health 48*: 21–28.

Dryden W (2019). *Single-Session Therapy: 100 key points and techniques.* Abingdon: Routledge.

Ellis A (1989). Using rational-emotive therapy (RET) as crisis intervention: a single session with a suicidal client. *Individual Psychology 45*: 75–81.

Erstling SS, Devlin J (1989). The single-session family interview. *Journal of Family Practice 28*: 556-560.

Gawrysiak, M, Nicholas C, Hopko DR (2009). Behavioral activation for moderately depressed university students: randomized controlled trial. *Journal of Counseling Psychology 56*: 468–475.

Green K, Correia T, Bobele M, Slive A (2011). The research case for walk-in single sessions. In: Slive A, Bobele M (eds). *When One Hour Is All You Have: effective therapy for walk-in clients*. Phoenix, AZ: Zeig, Tucker & Theisen (pp23–36).

Green S (2014). Horse sense: equine assisted single session consultations. In: Hoyt MF, Talmon M (eds). *Capturing the Moment: single session therapy and walk-in services*. Bethel, CT: Crown House Publishing (pp425–440).

Guthrie B (2018). Reflections on providing single-session therapy in post-disaster Haiti. In: Hoyt MF, Bobele M, Slive A, Young J, Talmon M (eds). *Single-Session Therapy by Walk-In or Appointment: administrative, clinical, and supervisory aspects of one-at-a-time services*. New York, NY: Routledge (pp. 303–317).

Harman R (1995). Gestalt therapy as brief therapy. *Gestalt Journal 18*: 77–85.

Harper-Jaques S (2018). Supervision and the single-session therapist: learnings from ten years of practice. In: Hoyt MF, Bobele M, Slive A, Young J, Talmon M (eds). *Single-Session Therapy by Walk-In or Appointment: administrative, clinical, and supervisory aspects of one-at-a-time services*. New York, NY: Routledge (pp. 334–346).

Howard KI, Kopta SM, Krause MS, Orlinsky DE (1986). The dose-effect relationship in psychotherapy. *American Psychologist 41*: 159–164.

Hoyt MF, Bobele M, Slive A, Young J, Talmon M (eds) (2018a). *Single-Session Therapy by Walk-In or Appointment: administrative, clinical, and supervisory aspects of one-at-a-time services*. New York, NY: Routledge.

Hoyt MF, Bobele M, Slive A, Young J, Talmon M (2018b). Single-session/one-at-a-time walk-in therapy. In: Hoyt MF, Bobele M, Slive A, Young J, Talmon M (eds). *Single-Session Therapy by Walk-In or Appointment: administrative, clinical, and supervisory aspects of one-at-a-time services*. New York, NY: Routledge (pp3–24).

Hoyt MF, Bobele M, Slive A, Young J, Talmon M (2018c). Walk-in and by-appointment single sessions now and in the future. In: Hoyt MF, Bobele M, Slive A, Young J, Talmon M (eds). *Single-Session Therapy by Walk-In or Appointment: administrative, clinical, and supervisory aspects of one-at-a-time services*. New York, NY: Routledge (pp. 369–379).

Hoyt MF, Talmon MF (eds) (2014a). *Capturing the moment: single session therapy and walk-in services*. Bethel, CT: Crown House Publishing.

Hoyt MF, Talmon MF (2014b). What the literature says: an annotated bibliography. In: Hoyt MF, Talmon M (eds). *Capturing the Moment: single-session therapy and walk-in services*. Bethel, CT: Crown House Publishing (pp487–516).

Hurn R (2005). Single-session therapy: planned success or unplanned failure? *Counselling Psychology Review 20*: 33–40.

Hymmen P, Stalker CA, Cait C-A (2013). The case for single-session therapy: does the empirical evidence support the increased prevalence of this service delivery model? *Journal of Mental Health 22*: 60–71.

Lamsal R, Stalker CA, Cait C-A, Riemer M, Horton S (2018). Cost-effectiveness analysis of single-session walk-in counselling. *Journal of Mental Health 27*: 560–566.

Littrell JM, Malia JA, Vanderwood M (1995). Single-session brief counselling in a high school. *Journal of Counseling and Development 73*: 451–458.

Marcus JD (1999). An Eriksonian approach to crack cocaine addiction: a single-session intervention. *Contemporary Hypnosis 16*: 95–102.

Miller JK, Slive A (2004). Breaking down the barriers to clinical service delivery: walk-in family therapy. *Journal of Marital & Family Therapy 30*: 95–103.

Miller WR (2000). Rediscovering fire: small interventions, large effects. *Psychology of Addictive Behaviours 14*: 6–18.

Perkins R (2006). The effectiveness of one session of therapy using a single-session therapy approach for children and adolescents with mental health problems. *Psychology and Psychotherapy: theory, research and practice 79*: 215–227.

Pitt T, Thomas O, Lindsay P, Hanton S, Bawden M (2015). Doing sport psychology briefly? A critical review of single session therapeutic approaches and their relevance to sport psychology. *International Review of Sport and Exercise Psychology 8*: 125–155.

Platt JJ, Mondellini D (2014). Single-session walk-in therapy for street robbery victims in Mexico City. In: Hoyt MF, Talmon M (eds) (2014). *Capturing the Moment: single session therapy and walk-in services*. Bethel, CT: Crown House Publishing (pp215–231).

Rodda SN, Lubman DI, Jackson AC, Dowling NA (2017). Improved outcomes following a single session web-based intervention for problem gambling. *Journal of Gambling Studies 33*: 283–299.

Rose S, Bisson J, Wessely S (2003). A systematic review of single-session psychological interventions ('debriefing') following trauma. *Psychotherapy and Psychosomatics 72*: 176–184.

Rosenbaum R, Hoyt MF, Talmon M (1990). The challenge of single-session therapies: creating pivotal moments. In: Wells RA, Giannetti VJ (eds). *Handbook of the Brief Psychotherapies*. New York, NY: Plenum Press (pp165-185).

Schleider JL, Weisz JR (2017). Little treatments, promising effects? Meta-analysis of single-session interventions for youth psychiatric problems. *Journal of the American Academy of Child & Adolescent Psychiatry 56*: 107-115.

Seligman MEP (1995). The effectiveness of psychotherapy: the consumer reports study. *American Psychologist 50*: 965-974.

Slaff B (1995). Thoughts on short-term and single-session therapy. In: Marohn RC, Feinstein SC (eds). *Adolescent Psychiatry: developmental and clinical studies: vol 20*. Hillsdale, NJ: Analytic Press (pp299-306).

Slive A, MacLaurin B, Oakander M, Amundson J (1995). Walk-in single sessions: a new paradigm in clinical service delivery. *Journal of Systemic Therapies 14*: 3-11.

Slive A, McElheran N, Lawson A (2008). How brief does it get? Walk-in single-session therapy. *Journal of Systemic Therapies 27*: 5-22.

Stacey K, Allison S, Dadds V, Roeger L, Wood A, Martin G (2001). Maintaining the gains: what worked in the year after brief family therapy. *Australian & New Zealand Journal of Family Therapy 22: 181-188*.

Talmon M (1990). *Single-Session Therapy: maximizing the effect of the first (and often only) therapeutic encounter*. San Francisco, CA: Jossey-Bass.

Ticho EA (1972). Termination of psychoanalysis: treatment goals, life goals. *Psychoanalytic Quarterly 41*: 315-333.

Young J, Rycroft P, Weir S (2014). Implementing single session therapy: practical wisdoms from down under. In: Hoyt MF, Talmon M (eds) (2014a). *Capturing the Moment: single session therapy and walk-in services*. Bethel, CT: Crown House Publishing (pp121-140).

Zlomke K, Davis III TE (2008). One-session treatment of specific phobias: a detailed description and review of treatment efficacy. *Behavior Therapy 39*: 207-223.

Index

W

Y

Z

The Primers in Counselling Series by PCCS Books

This best-selling series offers comprehensive descriptions of key counselling approaches and contexts in the 21st century. Accessible and concise, they are ideal for students seeking a theory bridge between introductory, intermediate and diploma courses or for comparative essays and integrative theory assignments.

The other primers in the series are:

The Person-Centred Counselling Primer – Pete Sanders
Paperback 9781898059806 – ebook 9781906254841

The Integrative Counselling Primer – Richard Worsley
Paperback 9781898059813 – ebook 9781906254902

The Experiential Counselling Primer – Mick Baker
Paperback 9781898059837

The Contact Work Primer: introduction to pre-therapy –
edited by Pete Sanders
Paperback 9781898059844

The Focusing-Oriented Counselling Primer –
Campbell Purton
Paperback 9781898059820 – ebook 9781906254889

The Psychodynamic Counselling Primer – Mavis Klein
Paperback 9781898059851 – ebook 9781906254896

The Cognitive Behavioural Counselling Primer –
Rhena Branch and Windy Dryden
Paperback 9781898059868 – ebook 9781906254919

The Existential Counselling Primer – Mick Cooper
Paperback 9781906254513 – ebook 9781906254858

The School-Based Counselling Primer – Katie McArthur
Paperback 9781906254780 – ebook 9781910919224

Discounted prices and free UK P&P – www.pccs-books.co.uk